Deluxe Diabetes Food & Blood Sugar Journal

By Habitually Healthy Publishing

Your greatest wealth is your health.

Habitually Healthy Publishing offers the information in this journal for informational purposes only and makes no claims regards the interpretation or utilization of any information in the journal.

All rights are reserved, including the right to reproduce this journal in whole, or any portion, in any form.

www.habitually-healthy.com

> **"STRIVE FOR PROGRESS NOT PERFECTION."**

DEDICATION

This book is journal is dedicated to you.

For taking the first small step and deciding to be just that little bit better.

CONTENTS

Introduction 6
- Journaling Works 9
- Journal Overview 11
  - Four-Step Plan for Your Success 11
- Making your diabetes diet easier, faster and more effective –online guides 12

Step 1 – Setting intentions 16
- Personal Goals 17
- Daily Food Targets 20

Step 2 – Tracking Food 24
- Weekly Preparation 25
- How This Book Works 26
- Notes on Completing the Diary 30
- Daily Tracking
  - Month 1 34
  - Month 2 98
  - Month 3 162

Contents

Step 3 – Review **225**
- Before and After 226
- Tracking Charts 228
- Weekly Progress Chart 229

Step 4 - Celebrate **236**
- 3-Month Target Achieved 237

Appendix **239**
- Exercise Reference Guide 240
- Frequently Eaten Foods 242
- Recipe Notes 244

INTRODUCTION

A study of nearly 1,700 participants shows that keeping a food diary can double a person's weight-loss[1].
—*Kaiser Permanente's Center for Health Research*

We have often read forums, spoken with friends, and received emails from people on a diabetes diet stating they lost weight, gained better control over their blood glucose levels and overall felt much better but struggled with maintaining their *discipline and maintaining it over a long term*. We knew the traditional advice wasn't enough. "Try harder", "eat fewer calories", "exercise more", "remove all sugars from your diet", "try raspberry ketones", and so on was either outdated, did not work, or was just not helpful.

We started to look at the science behind motivation, discipline, and weight loss. Through our research, it became clear that a journal would be the answer. However, we did not want to create just "another way to track calories and blood glucose" we wanted to create a journal to support you fully.

ROUND PEGS AND SQUARE HOLES

Trying to use a normal food diary on the diabetes diet is like trying to put a round peg in a square hole.

It just doesn't fit. The design of generic food journals is typically created for a standard American diet with conventional advice for general health. With this in mind, we realized that, although all the information we need to start a diabetes diet is already at

---

[1] https://www.sciencedaily.com/releases/2008/07/080708080738.htm

our fingertips, we are missing one vital tool: a journal that caters specifically to the diabetes diet and lifestyle.

A food journal is not just about losing weight (although this can be nice), it is also how you can take control of your blood glucose levels. Tracking your food and your body's reaction to it, helps you and your doctor to alter your diet and have long term control over your health.

This was our inspiration in creating the Deluxe Diabetes journal. A beautifully crafted planner, tailored specifically for you on your diabetes diet journey. It includes the key component measures of diabetes dieting and all the advice and encouragement you will need on your journey.

NOT JUST A FOOD JOURNAL

We looked at the science of motivation and included the best tools and strategies to ensure you are motivated and keep progressing toward your health goals.

By supporting you in your progression and recording your daily food intake and exercise routine, the accountability and practice of writing everything down will help motivate you to focus on and achieve your goals. You will be inspired to remain disciplined and maintain good habits.

While the journal is tailored for the diabetes diet, please feel free to use as much or as little of the diary as you like. It is designed to be flexible depending on your goals and preferences. Our goal was to design an appealing and accessible product, created specifically to meet your needs.

Weight-loss and health success takes keeping track of everything you are putting in your body, having a plan and implementing it, and using the science of motivation – not just willpower – to achieve your goals daily.

That's where this journal completes the puzzle. Use this diary alongside a diabetes diet and you will double your chances of succeeding. Whether you are just starting a diet, trying to break through a plateau, or just want to try something different, you will surely find the help you need in these pages.

JOURNALING WORKS

Researchers (and marketers) have known for a long time that the majority of our decisions are subconscious. One study concludes that "your brain makes up its mind up to 10 seconds before you realize it."[2] Unfortunately, our unconscious decisions tend not to be what is best for us.

When you see that chocolate donut, your brain has already decided it wants it and it is very hard to fight that impulse.

We need to take our (negative) eating and exercising habits off autopilot and be aware of our decision making. We can then rewire our brain to make the positive habits our new autopilot. This is the power of a journal.

Simply having a journal makes us aware of our habits by:

- Creating awareness of current eating patterns
- Offering accountability to yourself for your goals
- Establishing new positive habits
- Keeping you motivated with tangible, documented, and positive results from your efforts.

---

[2] https://www.relationshipscoach.co.uk/blog/research-shows-our-subconscious-mind-makes-our-decisions-for-us/

"THERE IS NO ONE **GIANT STEP** THAT DOES IT. IT'S LOTS OF **LITTLE STEPS**"

Introduction

JOURNAL OVERVIEW

FOUR-STEP PLAN FOR YOUR SUCCESS

Step 1: Set Goals – Create Motivation

Setting realistic goals and stating why you want to achieve them will help you get started and keep going when it gets tough.

Step 2: Take Action – Write It Down

Track your food, beverage, and exercise regimen so you stay disciplined and accountable for your goals. Aside from just recording your food, reaffirming your goals, reviewing the previous week and motivational quotes help to keep you on track.

Step 3: Review Your Progress

Check your progress periodically and take pride in your accomplishments to reinforce your new positive eating habits. In this section, you will find ways to:

- Record your before and after measurements
- Visually track your progress on line charts (using any measurement you want)

Step 4: Celebrate

Commemorate all the small and big wins so you can stay motivated and continue moving toward your goals.

MAKING THE DIABETES DIET EASIER, FASTER, AND MORE EFFECTIVE – ONLINE DOWNLOADABLE GUIDES

Inside this section are invaluable guides that will make your diabetes diet lifestyle easier. Learn how to change your life in 5 seconds, use intermittent fasting for greater results and some great meal ideas. Want to know the best day to start a diet (according to science), you'll find that here too.

Appendix

This section includes an abundance of useful information and a place for your own notes. It contains a

- guide to calories burned by common exercise.
- pages to record your most frequent food nutritional information.
- store your favorite recipes.

> **"I BELIEVE THAT THE GREATEST GIFT YOU CAN GIVE YOUR FAMILY AND THE WORLD IS A HEALTHY YOU"**
>
> — JOYCE MEYER

MAKING WEIGHT-LOSS EASIER, FASTER AND MORE EFFECTIVE ONLINE GUIDES

This an online section intended to make your lifestyle on the diabetic diet that little bit easier. Plus, it's about helping you overcome some key challenges you might find along the way, from just starting to "tricking" yourself into losing more weight – all backed by science.

These are intended to be "extras" and are not essential. We would recommend having a read and see if any ideas jump out at you or come back to this section if you are having a specific problem, such as trying to motivate yourself to start.

Visit the below site to download your guide.
www.habitually-healthy.com/diabetic-hacks

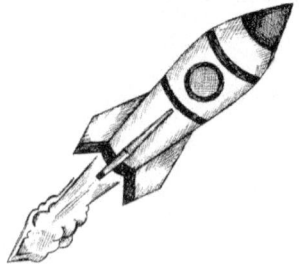

CONTENTS FOR ONLINE GUIDES

Favorite online recipe sources

Looking for some yummy meal ideas?
How about these to get started.

5 seconds to change your life

This brilliant 5 second rule has changed our lives,
worth a 60 second read.

Intermittent Fasting

This process can speed up your results or overcome plateaus.
Find out all of the what's, how's, whys, and what nots.

Using the Placebo Effect to Boost Weight-Loss

With this little Jedi mind trick, you might be able to speed up
your results – and it is backed up by science.

Best Day to Start a Diet (according to science)

Science declares that "today" is not necessarily the best day to
start a diet. Improve your chances with these suggestions.

Lifestyle Hacks

Sometimes, it is the little things which
can make a big difference.
These handy tips could make your life easier.

STEP 1
SETTING INTENTIONS

Simply writing your food down is not enough. Prepare and motivate yourself and take the 7-day challenge to keep on track.

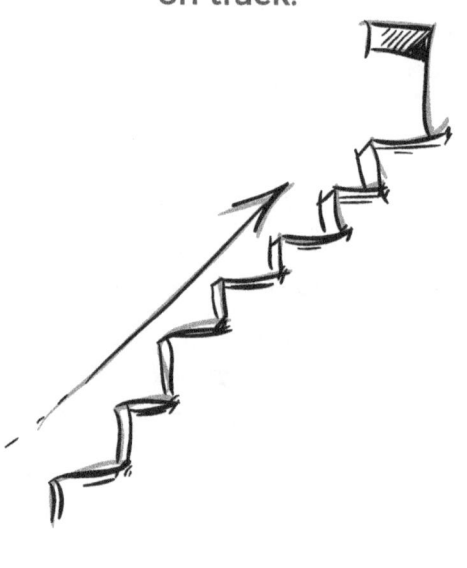

PERSONAL GOALS

"(S)he who has a why to live for can bear almost anyhow."
— *Friedrich Nietzsche*

Having a goal and a strong "why" will keep you motivated when it gets hard.

The goal doesn't have to be to lose X number of pounds or bring down your long-term glucose levels to Y. It could be instead simply to complete three months of the diary. What is of *greater importance is your "why"* – your reason for wanting to achieve the goal.

Wanting to lose weight just for the sake of losing weight is not usually motivating enough. You may wish to lose weight for health reasons, to be able to play with your new nephew, to attend a wedding that is coming up, or perhaps to feel more confident in yourself. There may be a small reward involved like a vacation, massage, or some new clothes.

It is your reason that will keep you motivated. Make sure it is strong.

Goal: _____

_____

I will achieve this by: _____

_____

I will achieve this because: _____

_____

_____

TIPS FOR GOAL SETTING

- **Make it specific.** For example, if you want to lose weight, write, "Lose 10 pounds within next 4 weeks." If you are working specifically on your physique, write "Lose 2 inches in the next six weeks."
- **Use the affirmative.** Rather than "I want to lose 10 pounds," write "I will lose 10 pounds ...." Such statements have proven to have subtle positive effects on your mind.
- **Make it realistic.** Losing 50 pounds in a week is not reasonable and will lead to disappointment. Make it a "Goldilocks" goal – not too easy and not too hard.
- **Set a deadline.** Having an end point of time involved makes the goal more real. This journal is for three months, so consider that as a deadline.

Step 1 – Setting Intentions

THREE MONTHS FROM NOW, YOU WILL THANK YOURSELF.

DAILY FOOD TARGETS

Record your daily targets for food and exercise.

Unfortunately, there is no 'standard' guide to how many grams of fats, carbs and proteins you should take. In a 2014 paper by the NCBI (Nutritional Recommendations for Individuals with Diabetes) stated:

> 'the best mix of carbohydrate, protein, and fat depends on the individual metabolic goals and preferences of the person with diabetes. It's most important to ensure that total calories are kept in mind for weight loss or maintenance'.[3]

Ideally, consult your doctor or nutritionist for a personalized recommended macronutrient intake. If this is not possible, we can use online calculators to which consider variables, such as age, gender, daily activity, and so on. I would recommend using the calculator at healthy-ojas, which considers a range of factors including your lifestyle and weight-loss targets.

http://healthy-ojas.com/calculator/macronutrient-calculator.html

Revisit this calculator monthly. If you lose weight, your targets will change accordingly.

Calories: _____ Fats: _____ Carbs: _____

Total Sugar: _____ Added Sugar: _____

Fiber: _____ Protein: _____

---

[3] https://www.ncbi.nlm.nih.gov/books/NBK279012/

Step 1 – Setting Intentions

Not everyone needs to go to the gym to get the benefits of exercise. One study claims walking just 20 minutes a day cuts your risk of premature death by almost one-third.[4]

Physical activity target

Week: _____

Day: _____

Quantity / Time: _____

See the end of the book for a "calories burned by exercise" reference guide.

---

[4] http://www.cam.ac.uk/research/news/lack-of-exercise-responsible-for-twice- as-many-deaths-as-obesity

7-DAY CHALLENGE

I am confident that if you can complete this diary for just seven days, then you can complete it for 14 days. If you can complete 14 days, then you can complete 30 days. After 30 days, you can then go on to 60 days and then 90 days.

If you can complete 90 days, then you will have achieved almost any health goal you have set.

The first seven days are the hardest, but we have a few tools to keep you going. In this book, you will find sections that:

- **Motivate you** – Set your intentions with your goals and reasons why
- **Keep you disciplined** – Set daily targets to stay on track
- **Inspire you** – Make some dishes from recipe ideas that make you feel creative. Find our favorite places to find recipes in the downloadable guide.
- **Make it fun** – This journal has been designed to make your transition into the diabetic lifestyle a fun process

THE CHALLENGE

If you can do these simple tasks every day for seven days, you will be well on your way to achieving your goals:

1. **Review your goals and reasons every morning.**
   – Keep yourself motivated and keep your goals in mind.
2. **Take your diary (and pen) everywhere you go.**
   – Hold yourself accountable everywhere with this journal.
3. **Write everything down.** Fill in this diary anytime you eat or drink something immediately when you consume it.
4. **Review it at the end of every day.** Review your accomplishments each day and celebrate every step closer to your goals.
5. **Celebrate on day seven.** At the end of the week, celebrate that you completed the challenge (fat bombs are particularly good for this).

This entire process should take you no longer than 30 minutes every day. That is 3½ hours out of 168 in your entire week (or 2 percent of your time). It takes just a small-time commitment to achieve your big goals..

STEP 2
TRACKING FOOD

This is where 'the rubber meets the road', and you put in the hard work to track your food intake.

You'll also find best practices, motivation and celebrations in the section to help you on your journey.

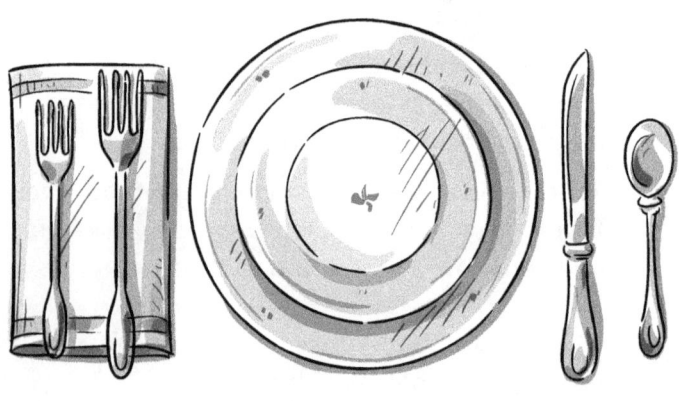

WEEKLY PREPARATION

MAKING DECISIONS THE EASY WAY

In the report 'What You Need To Know About Willpower: The Psychological Science of Self-control',[5] the American Psychological Association states "A growing body of research shows that resisting repeated temptations takes a mental toll." Some experts liken willpower to a muscle that can get fatigued from overuse.

This is similar to gas in a tank, the more decisions you make during a day, the more decision fatigued you become. Rest and recuperation then replenishes your tank. This explains why you are more likely to break a diet towards the end of the day than the start of a day.

HOW TO STAY ON TRACK WHEN DECISION MAKING FATIGUE OCCURS

As your day progresses, your "tank" will deplete, and you will begin to make habitual decisions, which at the start will likely be poor food (whatever is closest at hand).

Plan out your days and weeks in advance and "make the decision" ahead of time. Plan your meals and get snacks ready.

Attempt to establish a habit of planning and preparing meals either on the weekend or the night before and your chances of success will increase further.

---

[5] http://www.apa.org/helpcenter/willpower.aspx

HOW THIS BOOK WORKS - RECORDING FOOD

Over the next few pages, the daily food log will be introduced, with explanations and examples of how to use each section.

1 Date and Day - Circle the day and enter the date. Include a day number if you wish.

2 Food Tracking - Contains all of the required details for your diet. If possible, try and plan it out the day before – this will help to resist urges for "convenient snacks." Enter the time of the food, which can help you to notice trends.

3 Water - Try to consume the recommended eight 8-ounce glasses of water. Cross them out as you drink each glass.

Step 2 – Tracking Food

Date: Day 1 – 1st January   Mon. Tue. Wed. Thur. Fri. (Sat.) Sun.

BREAKFAST	Amount	Cal.	Fat gm	Carb. gm	Fiber gm	Sugar gm	Added sugar gm	Protein gm
Zucchini	½	16	0	3	1			1
Salmon fillet	1 fillet	241	14					28
Green onions	½ cup	16	0	2	2			
Coconut oil	1 tbsp	120	14					
Crumbled feta	½ cup	198	16	3				10
⏲ midday TOTAL		591	44	8	3			39

Insulin: Pre-sugar level: Post sugar level:

SNACK	Amount	Cal.	Fat gm	Carb. gm	Fiber gm	Sugar gm	Added sugar gm	Protein gm
Bulletproof coffee	1 cup	228	26			3	3	

⏲ 2pm   TOTAL

Insulin: Pre-sugar level: Post sugar level:

LUNCH	Amount	Cal.	Fat gm	Carb. gm	Fiber gm	Sugar gm	Added sugar gm	Protein gm
Pesto Spaghetti	1 serve	521	45	2	1	2	2	29

⏲ 3pm   TOTAL

Insulin: Pre-sugar level: Post sugar level:

SNACK	Amount	Cal.	Fat gm	Carb. gm	Fiber gm	Sugar gm	Added sugar gm	Protein gm
Hummus + cucumber	50g	125	9	5	2	5	2	5

⏲ 6pm   TOTAL

Insulin: Pre-sugar level: Post sugar level:

✗ ✗ ✗ ✗ 🥛 🥛 🥛 🥛   8 oz

4 Daily Total and Target - Sum your daily total calories and macronutrients. You may not require them all – such as fiber.

Daily target - Enter your daily targets for calories and macronutrients. Compare them to your actual totals at the end of the day. How close were they?

5 Ketone Levels – If you are following a keto or low carb diet, this gauge is for recording your ketone levels. Visually, it indicates whether you are in ketosis (0- 5-3.0mm) within the large markers. Mark off and record your levels. There is also a daily tracking chart in the reference section for a visual record over time.

6 Recording Exercise - Recording even the smallest exercise is beneficial as it shows your improvement and is motivating to reflect on. In the reference section is a guide to calories burned by common exercises.

7 Vitamins, Supplements, and Medications- List any supplements or medicine you are taking. This can be useful as a reminder or as a record to look back on later.

8 How was today - Record small wins, how you felt, and what you might do better tomorrow (set a positive intent).

Step 2 – Tracking Food

DINNER	Amount	Cal.	Fat gm	Carb. gm	Fiber gm	Sugar gm	Added sugar gm	Protein gm
chicken breast	1	231	5					43
avocado	½ med	70	7	4	1	3		
Pesto – homemade!	2 tsp	12	1					
🕐 7pm TOTAL		313	13	4	1	3		43

Insulin: Pre-sugar level: Post sugar level:

SNACK	Amount	Cal.	Fat gm	Carb. gm	Fiber gm	Sugar gm	Added sugar gm	Protein gm
🕐 8pm TOTAL								

Insulin: Pre-sugar level: Post sugar level:

Daily Total		1613	128	14	5	9		11
Daily Target		1500	133	20		20		58

(4)

(5) Ketone Levels (mM)

0   0.5   1.0   1.5   2.~~0~~   2.5   3.0   5.0+   *2.4*

(7) Vitamins / Supplements / Meds.

Description	Qty	
Potassium	1	1
Multi vitamin	1	

(6) Exercise notes

What ____walked to store____

Duration ____30 mins____

Calories Burned ____160____

(8) How was today?

Felt good today. Macros were good (bit too much protein... will watch it tomorrow. Overall happy with day!

😟   😔   😐   🙂   **(😄)**

NOTES ON COMPLETING THE DIARY

- **Don't skip the front section.** The "Personal Goals" section will help keep you motivated so you can maintain your discipline.
- **Be as accurate as possible.** It is easy to try and "guess" portions. Try to record it when you consume it.
- **Include all the extras.** That coffee you picked up while you were out or that little nibble on the cookie – they all count! Write it down.
- **Don't beat yourself up over mistakes.** Know that you will slip up but don't give yourself a hard time. Write it down and learn from it moving forward.
- **Review your diary.** Reviewing your diary on a weekly basis will reveal progression and eating patterns, which will help to keep you motivated.
- **Keep it with you,** everywhere. Recording your food and drink "in the moment" is always more preferable than trying to remember something later. We tend to forget or distort what we actually consumed. It's best to write it down immediately so you don't have to rely on your memory.
- **Be as detailed as you want to be.** This diary provides all the information you could need but it should feel easy and not like a chore when completing the meals.
- **Cook at home.** Try cooking at home as much as possible, as it makes recording your food that much easier.
- **Connect with the tracking.** Try not to 'just write' your food down, but get a 'sense' for what 400 calories or you total daily calorie count physically looks like. It will help you feel how much food you need to 'be full'. This is intuitive eating and could mean no longer tracking food (if you wish).

REAFFIRMING COMMITMENT

Studies have shown "you become 42% more likely to achieve your goals and dreams, simply by writing them down on a regular basis".[6]

It is the start of a new week, so reaffirm your commitment to your goals and increase your chances of success. When writing your goals 'feel' they are coming true and ensure your reasons for wanting the goal are strong.

Goal: _____

_____

I will achieve this by: _____

_____

I will achieve this because: _____

_____

_____

_____

_____

---

[6] https://www.huffingtonpost.com/marymorrissey/the-power-of-writing-down_b_12002348.html

NOW IT IS YOUR TURN.

Focus on the single step / day in front of you.

Before starting your first day, remember:

Decide

Commit

Prepare

Take consistent positive action

"YOU DO NOT HAVE TO SEE THE WHOLE STAIRCASE, JUST TAKE THE FIRST STEP"

WEEK OF ____

Date:				Mon.	Tue.	Wed.	Thur.	Fri.	Sat.	Sun.
BREAKFAST		Amount	Cal.	Fat gm	Carb. gm	Fiber gm	Sugar gm	Added sugar gm	Protein gm
	TOTAL									
Insulin:	Pre-sugar level:			Post sugar level:						

SNACK		Amount	Cal.	Fat gm	Carb. gm	Fiber gm	Sugar gm	Added sugar gm	Protein gm
	TOTAL								
Insulin:	Pre-sugar level:		Post sugar level:						

LUNCH		Amount	Cal.	Fat gm	Carb. gm	Fiber gm	Sugar gm	Added sugar gm	Protein gm
	TOTAL								
Insulin:	Pre-sugar level:		Post sugar level:						

SNACK		Amount	Cal.	Fat gm	Carb. gm	Fiber gm	Sugar gm	Added sugar gm	Protein gm
	TOTAL								
Insulin:	Pre-sugar level:		Post sugar level:						

        8 oz

Step 2 – Tracking Food

DINNER	Amount	Cal.	Fat gm	Carb. gm	Fiber gm	Sugar gm	Added sugar gm	Protein gm
TOTAL								

Insulin: _____ Pre-sugar level: _____ Post sugar level: _____

SNACK	Amount	Cal.	Fat gm	Carb. gm	Fiber gm	Sugar gm	Added sugar gm	Protein gm
TOTAL								

Insulin: _____ Pre-sugar level: _____ Post sugar level: _____

| Daily Total | | | | | | | | |
| Daily Target | | | | | | | | |

Ketone Levels (mM)

|—|—|—|—|—|—|—|
0   0.5 1.0 1.5 2.0 2.5 3.0   5.0+

Exercise notes

What _____

Duration _____

Calories Burned _____

Vitamins / Supplements / Meds.

Description	Qty

How was today?

_____

_____

DAILY

Date: _____ Mon. Tue. Wed. Thur. Fri. Sat. Sun.

BREAKFAST	Amount	Cal.	Fat gm	Carb. gm	Fiber gm	Sugar gm	Added sugar gm	Protein gm
TOTAL								

Insulin: _____ Pre-sugar level: _____ Post sugar level: _____

SNACK	Amount	Cal.	Fat gm	Carb. gm	Fiber gm	Sugar gm	Added sugar gm	Protein gm
TOTAL								

Insulin: _____ Pre-sugar level: _____ Post sugar level: _____

LUNCH	Amount	Cal.	Fat gm	Carb. gm	Fiber gm	Sugar gm	Added sugar gm	Protein gm
TOTAL								

Insulin: _____ Pre-sugar level: _____ Post sugar level: _____

SNACK	Amount	Cal.	Fat gm	Carb. gm	Fiber gm	Sugar gm	Added sugar gm	Protein gm
TOTAL								

Insulin: _____ Pre-sugar level: _____ Post sugar level: _____

         8 oz

Step 2 – Tracking Food

DINNER	Amount	Cal.	Fat gm	Carb. gm	Fiber gm	Sugar gm	Added sugar gm	Protein gm
TOTAL								

Insulin: _____ Pre-sugar level: _____ Post sugar level: _____

SNACK	Amount	Cal.	Fat gm	Carb. gm	Fiber gm	Sugar gm	Added sugar gm	Protein gm
TOTAL								

Insulin: _____ Pre-sugar level: _____ Post sugar level: _____

| Daily Total | | | | | | | | |
| Daily Target | | | | | | | | |

Ketone Levels (mM)

0   0.5   1.0   1.5   2.0   2.5   3.0   5.0+

Exercise notes

What _____

Duration _____

Calories Burned _____

Vitamins / Supplements / Meds.

Description	Qty

How was today?

_____

_____

_____

DAILY

Date: Mon.   Tue.   Wed.   Thur.   Fri.   Sat.   Sun.

BREAKFAST	Amount	Cal.	Fat gm	Carb. gm	Fiber gm	Sugar gm	Added sugar gm	Protein gm
	TOTAL							

Insulin: Pre-sugar level: Post sugar level:

SNACK	Amount	Cal.	Fat gm	Carb. gm	Fiber gm	Sugar gm	Added sugar gm	Protein gm
	TOTAL							

Insulin: Pre-sugar level: Post sugar level:

LUNCH	Amount	Cal.	Fat gm	Carb. gm	Fiber gm	Sugar gm	Added sugar gm	Protein gm
	TOTAL							

Insulin: Pre-sugar level: Post sugar level:

SNACK	Amount	Cal.	Fat gm	Carb. gm	Fiber gm	Sugar gm	Added sugar gm	Protein gm
	TOTAL							

Insulin: Pre-sugar level: Post sugar level:

          8 oz

Step 2 – Tracking Food

DINNER	Amount	Cal.	Fat gm	Carb. gm	Fiber gm	Sugar gm	Added sugar gm	Protein gm
TOTAL								

Insulin: _____ Pre-sugar level: _____ Post sugar level: _____

SNACK	Amount	Cal.	Fat gm	Carb. gm	Fiber gm	Sugar gm	Added sugar gm	Protein gm
TOTAL								

Insulin: _____ Pre-sugar level: _____ Post sugar level: _____

| Daily Total | | | | | | | | |
| Daily Target | | | | | | | | |

Ketone Levels (mM)

|—|—|—|—|—|—|—|
| 0 | 0.5 | 1.0 | 1.5 | 2.0 | 2.5 | 3.0 | 5.0+ |

Exercise notes

What _____

Duration _____

Calories Burned _____

Vitamins / Supplements / Meds.

Description	Qty

How was today?

_____

_____

DAILY

Date: Mon. Tue. Wed. Thur. Fri. Sat. Sun.

BREAKFAST	Amount	Cal.	Fat gm	Carb. gm	Fiber gm	Sugar gm	Added sugar gm	Protein gm
TOTAL								

Insulin: _____ Pre-sugar level: _____ Post sugar level: _____

SNACK	Amount	Cal.	Fat gm	Carb. gm	Fiber gm	Sugar gm	Added sugar gm	Protein gm
TOTAL								

Insulin: _____ Pre-sugar level: _____ Post sugar level: _____

LUNCH	Amount	Cal.	Fat gm	Carb. gm	Fiber gm	Sugar gm	Added sugar gm	Protein gm
TOTAL								

Insulin: _____ Pre-sugar level: _____ Post sugar level: _____

SNACK	Amount	Cal.	Fat gm	Carb. gm	Fiber gm	Sugar gm	Added sugar gm	Protein gm
TOTAL								

Insulin: _____ Pre-sugar level: _____ Post sugar level: _____

         8 oz

Step 2 – Tracking Food

DINNER	Amount	Cal.	Fat gm	Carb. gm	Fiber gm	Sugar gm	Added sugar gm	Protein gm
TOTAL								

Insulin: _____ Pre-sugar level: _____ Post sugar level: _____

SNACK	Amount	Cal.	Fat gm	Carb. gm	Fiber gm	Sugar gm	Added sugar gm	Protein gm
TOTAL								

Insulin: _____ Pre-sugar level: _____ Post sugar level: _____

| Daily Total | | | | | | | | |
| Daily Target | | | | | | | | |

Ketone Levels (mM)

|—|—|—|—|—|—|—|
0   0.5   1.0   1.5   2.0   2.5   3.0   5.0+

Exercise notes

What _____

Duration _____

Calories Burned _____

Vitamins / Supplements / Meds.

Description	Qty

How was today?

_____

_____

_____

DAILY

Date: _____   Mon. Tue. Wed. Thur. Fri. Sat. Sun.

BREAKFAST	Amount	Cal.	Fat gm	Carb. gm	Fiber gm	Sugar gm	Added sugar gm	Protein gm
🕒 TOTAL								

Insulin: _____   Pre-sugar level: _____   Post sugar level: _____

SNACK	Amount	Cal.	Fat gm	Carb. gm	Fiber gm	Sugar gm	Added sugar gm	Protein gm
🕒 TOTAL								

Insulin: _____   Pre-sugar level: _____   Post sugar level: _____

LUNCH	Amount	Cal.	Fat gm	Carb. gm	Fiber gm	Sugar gm	Added sugar gm	Protein gm
🕒 TOTAL								

Insulin: _____   Pre-sugar level: _____   Post sugar level: _____

SNACK	Amount	Cal.	Fat gm	Carb. gm	Fiber gm	Sugar gm	Added sugar gm	Protein gm
🕒 TOTAL								

Insulin: _____   Pre-sugar level: _____   Post sugar level: _____

         8 oz

Step 2 – Tracking Food

DINNER	Amount	Cal.	Fat gm	Carb. gm	Fiber gm	Sugar gm	Added sugar gm	Protein gm
TOTAL								

Insulin: _____ Pre-sugar level: _____ Post sugar level: _____

SNACK	Amount	Cal.	Fat gm	Carb. gm	Fiber gm	Sugar gm	Added sugar gm	Protein gm
TOTAL								

Insulin: _____ Pre-sugar level: _____ Post sugar level: _____

| Daily Total | | | | | | | | |
| Daily Target | | | | | | | | |

Ketone Levels (mM)

0 0.5 1.0 1.5 2.0 2.5 3.0 5.0+

Exercise notes

What _____

Duration _____

Calories Burned _____

Vitamins / Supplements / Meds.

Description	Qty

How was today?

_____

_____

_____

DAILY

Date: Mon. Tue. Wed. Thur. Fri. Sat. Sun.

BREAKFAST	Amount	Cal.	Fat gm	Carb. gm	Fiber gm	Sugar gm	Added sugar gm	Protein gm
🕐 TOTAL								

Insulin: Pre-sugar level: Post sugar level:

SNACK	Amount	Cal.	Fat gm	Carb. gm	Fiber gm	Sugar gm	Added sugar gm	Protein gm
🕐 TOTAL								

Insulin: Pre-sugar level: Post sugar level:

LUNCH	Amount	Cal.	Fat gm	Carb. gm	Fiber gm	Sugar gm	Added sugar gm	Protein gm
🕐 TOTAL								

Insulin: Pre-sugar level: Post sugar level:

SNACK	Amount	Cal.	Fat gm	Carb. gm	Fiber gm	Sugar gm	Added sugar gm	Protein gm
🕐 TOTAL								

Insulin: Pre-sugar level: Post sugar level:

   8 oz

Step 2 – Tracking Food

DINNER	Amount	Cal.	Fat gm	Carb. gm	Fiber gm	Sugar gm	Added sugar gm	Protein gm
TOTAL								

Insulin: _____ Pre-sugar level: _____ Post sugar level: _____

SNACK	Amount	Cal.	Fat gm	Carb. gm	Fiber gm	Sugar gm	Added sugar gm	Protein gm
TOTAL								

Insulin: _____ Pre-sugar level: _____ Post sugar level: _____

| Daily Total | | | | | | | | |
| Daily Target | | | | | | | | |

Ketone Levels (mM)

0   0.5   1.0   1.5   2.0   2.5   3.0   5.0+

Exercise notes

What _____

Duration _____

Calories Burned _____

Vitamins / Supplements / Meds.

Description	Qty

How was today?

_____

_____

DAILY

Date: _____   Mon.   Tue.   Wed.   Thur.   Fri.   Sat.   Sun.

BREAKFAST	Amount	Cal.	Fat gm	Carb. gm	Fiber gm	Sugar gm	Added sugar gm	Protein gm
TOTAL								

Insulin: _____   Pre-sugar level: _____   Post sugar level: _____

SNACK	Amount	Cal.	Fat gm	Carb. gm	Fiber gm	Sugar gm	Added sugar gm	Protein gm
TOTAL								

Insulin: _____   Pre-sugar level: _____   Post sugar level: _____

LUNCH	Amount	Cal.	Fat gm	Carb. gm	Fiber gm	Sugar gm	Added sugar gm	Protein gm
TOTAL								

Insulin: _____   Pre-sugar level: _____   Post sugar level: _____

SNACK	Amount	Cal.	Fat gm	Carb. gm	Fiber gm	Sugar gm	Added sugar gm	Protein gm
TOTAL								

Insulin: _____   Pre-sugar level: _____   Post sugar level: _____

         8 oz

Step 2 – Tracking Food

DINNER	Amount	Cal.	Fat gm	Carb. gm	Fiber gm	Sugar gm	Added sugar gm	Protein gm
TOTAL								

Insulin: _____ Pre-sugar level: _____ Post sugar level: _____

SNACK	Amount	Cal.	Fat gm	Carb. gm	Fiber gm	Sugar gm	Added sugar gm	Protein gm
TOTAL								

Insulin: _____ Pre-sugar level: _____ Post sugar level: _____

| Daily Total | | | | | | | | |
| Daily Target | | | | | | | | |

Ketone Levels (mM)

├─┼─┼─┼─┼─┼─┤
0   0.5   1.0   1.5   2.0   2.5   3.0   5.0+

Exercise notes

What _____

Duration _____

Calories Burned _____

Vitamins / Supplements / Meds.

Description	Qty

How was today?

_____

_____

_____

WEEKLY WINS

What went well this week? What can I take forward to next week?

Making next week even better

What have you learned this week? What could have been better?

I seem to be eating worse in the afternoon and evenings, usually snacking on some chips or chocolate. There have been some very long meetings at work and there wasn't anything good in the room.

I am also struggling when out with friends, they always want to go to somewhere that I cannot eat well at.

What can you implement next week to ensure success?

I will buy some good snacks and take them to work, some nuts or perhaps make some of those yummy bars.

For my friends, I will suggest 'dinner parties' instead. If I propose the first one at my house, I can cook and also show them that being healthy can be delicious.

Do not forget to record any measurements you wish to track weekly in the reference section.

WEEKLY WINS

What went well this week? What can I take forward to next week?

Making next week even better

What have you learned this week? What could have been better?

_____
_____
_____
_____
_____
_____

What can you implement next week to ensure success?

_____
_____
_____
_____
_____
_____

Do not forget to record any measurements you wish to track weekly in the reference section.

WEEK OF ____

Date: _____   Mon. Tue. Wed. Thur. Fri. Sat. Sun.

BREAKFAST	Amount	Cal.	Fat gm	Carb. gm	Fiber gm	Sugar gm	Added sugar gm	Protein gm
TOTAL								

Insulin: _____ Pre-sugar level: _____ Post sugar level: _____

SNACK	Amount	Cal.	Fat gm	Carb. gm	Fiber gm	Sugar gm	Added sugar gm	Protein gm
TOTAL								

Insulin: _____ Pre-sugar level: _____ Post sugar level: _____

LUNCH	Amount	Cal.	Fat gm	Carb. gm	Fiber gm	Sugar gm	Added sugar gm	Protein gm
TOTAL								

Insulin: _____ Pre-sugar level: _____ Post sugar level: _____

SNACK	Amount	Cal.	Fat gm	Carb. gm	Fiber gm	Sugar gm	Added sugar gm	Protein gm
TOTAL								

Insulin: _____ Pre-sugar level: _____ Post sugar level: _____

         8 oz

Step 2 – Tracking Food

DINNER	Amount	Cal.	Fat gm	Carb. gm	Fiber gm	Sugar gm	Added sugar gm	Protein gm
TOTAL								

Insulin: _____ Pre-sugar level: _____ Post sugar level: _____

SNACK	Amount	Cal.	Fat gm	Carb. gm	Fiber gm	Sugar gm	Added sugar gm	Protein gm
TOTAL								

Insulin: _____ Pre-sugar level: _____ Post sugar level: _____

| Daily Total | | | | | | | | |
| Daily Target | | | | | | | | |

Ketone Levels (mM)

0   0.5   1.0   1.5   2.0   2.5   3.0   5.0+

Exercise notes

What _____

Duration _____

Calories Burned _____

Vitamins / Supplements / Meds.

Description	Qty

How was today?

_____

_____

DAILY

Date: Mon. Tue. Wed. Thur. Fri. Sat. Sun.

BREAKFAST	Amount	Cal.	Fat gm	Carb. gm	Fiber gm	Sugar gm	Added sugar gm	Protein gm
TOTAL								

Insulin: _____   Pre-sugar level: _____   Post sugar level: _____

SNACK	Amount	Cal.	Fat gm	Carb. gm	Fiber gm	Sugar gm	Added sugar gm	Protein gm
TOTAL								

Insulin: _____   Pre-sugar level: _____   Post sugar level: _____

LUNCH	Amount	Cal.	Fat gm	Carb. gm	Fiber gm	Sugar gm	Added sugar gm	Protein gm
TOTAL								

Insulin: _____   Pre-sugar level: _____   Post sugar level: _____

SNACK	Amount	Cal.	Fat gm	Carb. gm	Fiber gm	Sugar gm	Added sugar gm	Protein gm
TOTAL								

Insulin: _____   Pre-sugar level: _____   Post sugar level: _____

         8 oz

Step 2 – Tracking Food

DINNER	Amount	Cal.	Fat gm	Carb. gm	Fiber gm	Sugar gm	Added sugar gm	Protein gm
TOTAL								

Insulin: _____ Pre-sugar level: _____ Post sugar level: _____

SNACK	Amount	Cal.	Fat gm	Carb. gm	Fiber gm	Sugar gm	Added sugar gm	Protein gm
TOTAL								

Insulin: _____ Pre-sugar level: _____ Post sugar level: _____

| Daily Total | | | | | | | | |
| Daily Target | | | | | | | | |

Ketone Levels (mM)

|—+—+—+—+—+—+—|
0   0.5 1.0 1.5 2.0 2.5 3.0   5.0+

Exercise notes

What _____

Duration _____

Calories Burned _____

Vitamins / Supplements / Meds.

Description	Qty

How was today?

_____

_____

_____

DAILY

Date: Mon.   Tue.   Wed.   Thur.   Fri.   Sat.   Sun.

BREAKFAST	Amount	Cal.	Fat gm	Carb. gm	Fiber gm	Sugar gm	Added sugar gm	Protein gm
TOTAL								

Insulin: Pre-sugar level: Post sugar level:

SNACK	Amount	Cal.	Fat gm	Carb. gm	Fiber gm	Sugar gm	Added sugar gm	Protein gm
TOTAL								

Insulin: Pre-sugar level: Post sugar level:

LUNCH	Amount	Cal.	Fat gm	Carb. gm	Fiber gm	Sugar gm	Added sugar gm	Protein gm
TOTAL								

Insulin: Pre-sugar level: Post sugar level:

SNACK	Amount	Cal.	Fat gm	Carb. gm	Fiber gm	Sugar gm	Added sugar gm	Protein gm
TOTAL								

Insulin: Pre-sugar level: Post sugar level:

        8 oz

Step 2 – Tracking Food

DINNER	Amount	Cal.	Fat gm	Carb. gm	Fiber gm	Sugar gm	Added sugar gm	Protein gm
⏱ TOTAL								

Insulin: _____ Pre-sugar level: _____ Post sugar level: _____

SNACK	Amount	Cal.	Fat gm	Carb. gm	Fiber gm	Sugar gm	Added sugar gm	Protein gm
⏱ TOTAL								

Insulin: _____ Pre-sugar level: _____ Post sugar level: _____

| Daily Total | | | | | | | | |
| Daily Target | | | | | | | | |

Ketone Levels (mM)

| 0 | 0.5 | 1.0 | 1.5 | 2.0 | 2.5 | 3.0 | 5.0+ |

Exercise notes

What _____

Duration _____

Calories Burned _____

Vitamins / Supplements / Meds.

Description	Qty

How was today?

_____

_____

_____

DAILY

Date: _____   Mon. Tue. Wed. Thur. Fri. Sat. Sun.

BREAKFAST	Amount	Cal.	Fat gm	Carb. gm	Fiber gm	Sugar gm	Added sugar gm	Protein gm
🕐 TOTAL								

Insulin: _____   Pre-sugar level: _____   Post sugar level: _____

SNACK	Amount	Cal.	Fat gm	Carb. gm	Fiber gm	Sugar gm	Added sugar gm	Protein gm
🕐 TOTAL								

Insulin: _____   Pre-sugar level: _____   Post sugar level: _____

LUNCH	Amount	Cal.	Fat gm	Carb. gm	Fiber gm	Sugar gm	Added sugar gm	Protein gm
🕐 TOTAL								

Insulin: _____   Pre-sugar level: _____   Post sugar level: _____

SNACK	Amount	Cal.	Fat gm	Carb. gm	Fiber gm	Sugar gm	Added sugar gm	Protein gm
🕐 TOTAL								

Insulin: _____   Pre-sugar level: _____   Post sugar level: _____

8 oz

Step 2 – Tracking Food

DINNER	Amount	Cal.	Fat gm	Carb. gm	Fiber gm	Sugar gm	Added sugar gm	Protein gm
TOTAL								

Insulin: _____ Pre-sugar level: _____ Post sugar level: _____

SNACK	Amount	Cal.	Fat gm	Carb. gm	Fiber gm	Sugar gm	Added sugar gm	Protein gm
TOTAL								

Insulin: _____ Pre-sugar level: _____ Post sugar level: _____

| Daily Total | | | | | | | | |
| Daily Target | | | | | | | | |

Ketone Levels (mM)

0   0.5   1.0   1.5   2.0   2.5   3.0   5.0+

Exercise notes

What _____

Duration _____

Calories Burned _____

Vitamins / Supplements / Meds.

Description	Qty

How was today?

_____

_____

DAILY

Date: _____   Mon. Tue. Wed. Thur. Fri. Sat. Sun.

BREAKFAST	Amount	Cal.	Fat gm	Carb. gm	Fiber gm	Sugar gm	Added sugar gm	Protein gm
🕐 TOTAL								

Insulin: _____   Pre-sugar level: _____   Post sugar level: _____

SNACK	Amount	Cal.	Fat gm	Carb. gm	Fiber gm	Sugar gm	Added sugar gm	Protein gm
🕐 TOTAL								

Insulin: _____   Pre-sugar level: _____   Post sugar level: _____

LUNCH	Amount	Cal.	Fat gm	Carb. gm	Fiber gm	Sugar gm	Added sugar gm	Protein gm
🕐 TOTAL								

Insulin: _____   Pre-sugar level: _____   Post sugar level: _____

SNACK	Amount	Cal.	Fat gm	Carb. gm	Fiber gm	Sugar gm	Added sugar gm	Protein gm
🕐 TOTAL								

Insulin: _____   Pre-sugar level: _____   Post sugar level: _____

         8 oz

Step 2 – Tracking Food

DINNER	Amount	Cal.	Fat gm	Carb. gm	Fiber gm	Sugar gm	Added sugar gm	Protein gm
⏱ TOTAL								

Insulin: _____ Pre-sugar level: _____ Post sugar level: _____

SNACK	Amount	Cal.	Fat gm	Carb. gm	Fiber gm	Sugar gm	Added sugar gm	Protein gm
⏱ TOTAL								

Insulin: _____ Pre-sugar level: _____ Post sugar level: _____

| Daily Total | | | | | | | | |
| Daily Target | | | | | | | | |

Ketone Levels (mM)

|—|—|—|—|—|—|—|
0   0.5   1.0   1.5   2.0   2.5   3.0   5.0+

Vitamins / Supplements / Meds.

Description	Qty

Exercise notes

What _____

Duration _____

Calories Burned _____

How was today?

_____

_____

DAILY

Date: Mon. Tue. Wed. Thur. Fri. Sat. Sun.

BREAKFAST	Amount	Cal.	Fat gm	Carb. gm	Fiber gm	Sugar gm	Added sugar gm	Protein gm
TOTAL								

Insulin: ____   Pre-sugar level: ____   Post sugar level: ____

SNACK	Amount	Cal.	Fat gm	Carb. gm	Fiber gm	Sugar gm	Added sugar gm	Protein gm
TOTAL								

Insulin: ____   Pre-sugar level: ____   Post sugar level: ____

LUNCH	Amount	Cal.	Fat gm	Carb. gm	Fiber gm	Sugar gm	Added sugar gm	Protein gm
TOTAL								

Insulin: ____   Pre-sugar level: ____   Post sugar level: ____

SNACK	Amount	Cal.	Fat gm	Carb. gm	Fiber gm	Sugar gm	Added sugar gm	Protein gm
TOTAL								

Insulin: ____   Pre-sugar level: ____   Post sugar level: ____

         8 oz

Step 2 – Tracking Food

DINNER		Amount	Cal.	Fat gm	Carb. gm	Fiber gm	Sugar gm	Added sugar gm	Protein gm
⊙	TOTAL								
Insulin:	Pre-sugar level:		Post sugar level:						

SNACK		Amount	Cal.	Fat gm	Carb. gm	Fiber gm	Sugar gm	Added sugar gm	Protein gm
⊙	TOTAL								
Insulin:	Pre-sugar level:		Post sugar level:						
Daily Total									
Daily Target									

Ketone Levels (mM)

0 0.5 1.0 1.5 2.0 2.5 3.0 5.0+

Vitamins / Supplements / Meds.

Description	Qty

Exercise notes

What _____

Duration _____

Calories Burned _____

How was today?

_____

_____

DAILY

Date: Mon. Tue. Wed. Thur. Fri. Sat. Sun.

BREAKFAST	Amount	Cal.	Fat gm	Carb. gm	Fiber gm	Sugar gm	Added sugar gm	Protein gm
TOTAL								

Insulin: _____ Pre-sugar level: _____ Post sugar level: _____

SNACK	Amount	Cal.	Fat gm	Carb. gm	Fiber gm	Sugar gm	Added sugar gm	Protein gm
TOTAL								

Insulin: _____ Pre-sugar level: _____ Post sugar level: _____

LUNCH	Amount	Cal.	Fat gm	Carb. gm	Fiber gm	Sugar gm	Added sugar gm	Protein gm
TOTAL								

Insulin: _____ Pre-sugar level: _____ Post sugar level: _____

SNACK	Amount	Cal.	Fat gm	Carb. gm	Fiber gm	Sugar gm	Added sugar gm	Protein gm
TOTAL								

Insulin: _____ Pre-sugar level: _____ Post sugar level: _____

8 oz

Step 2 – Tracking Food

DINNER	Amount	Cal.	Fat gm	Carb. gm	Fiber gm	Sugar gm	Added sugar gm	Protein gm
TOTAL								

Insulin: _____ Pre-sugar level: _____ Post sugar level: _____

SNACK	Amount	Cal.	Fat gm	Carb. gm	Fiber gm	Sugar gm	Added sugar gm	Protein gm
TOTAL								

Insulin: _____ Pre-sugar level: _____ Post sugar level: _____

| Daily Total | | | | | | | | |
| Daily Target | | | | | | | | |

Ketone Levels (mM)

0   0.5   1.0   1.5   2.0   2.5   3.0   5.0+

Exercise notes

What _____

Duration _____

Calories Burned _____

Vitamins / Supplements / Meds.

Description	Qty

How was today?

_____
_____

WEEKLY WINS

What went well this week? What can I take forward to next week?

Making next week even better

What have you learned this week? What could have been better?

_____
_____
_____
_____
_____

What can you implement next week to ensure success?

_____
_____
_____
_____
_____

Do not forget to record any measurements you wish to track weekly in the reference section.

> **"THE BODY IS LIKE A PIANO, AND HAPPINESS IS LIKE MUSIC. IT IS NEEDFUL TO HAVE THE INSTRUMENT IN GOOD ORDER"**

WEEK OF ____

Date: Mon.   Tue.   Wed.   Thur.   Fri.   Sat.   Sun.

BREAKFAST	Amount	Cal.	Fat gm	Carb. gm	Fiber gm	Sugar gm	Added sugar gm	Protein gm
TOTAL								

Insulin: _____   Pre-sugar level: _____   Post sugar level: _____

SNACK	Amount	Cal.	Fat gm	Carb. gm	Fiber gm	Sugar gm	Added sugar gm	Protein gm
TOTAL								

Insulin: _____   Pre-sugar level: _____   Post sugar level: _____

LUNCH	Amount	Cal.	Fat gm	Carb. gm	Fiber gm	Sugar gm	Added sugar gm	Protein gm
TOTAL								

Insulin: _____   Pre-sugar level: _____   Post sugar level: _____

SNACK	Amount	Cal.	Fat gm	Carb. gm	Fiber gm	Sugar gm	Added sugar gm	Protein gm
TOTAL								

Insulin: _____   Pre-sugar level: _____   Post sugar level: _____

        8 oz

Step 2 – Tracking Food

DINNER		Amount	Cal.	Fat gm	Carb. gm	Fiber gm	Sugar gm	Added sugar gm	Protein gm
🕐	TOTAL								

Insulin: _____   Pre-sugar level: _____   Post sugar level: _____

SNACK		Amount	Cal.	Fat gm	Carb. gm	Fiber gm	Sugar gm	Added sugar gm	Protein gm
🕐	TOTAL								

Insulin: _____   Pre-sugar level: _____   Post sugar level: _____

| Daily Total | | | | | | | | |
| Daily Target | | | | | | | | |

Ketone Levels (mM)

0 — 0.5 — 1.0 — 1.5 — 2.0 — 2.5 — 3.0 — 5.0+

Exercise notes

What _____

Duration _____

Calories Burned _____

Vitamins / Supplements / Meds.

Description	Qty

How was today?

_____

_____

DAILY

Date: Mon. Tue. Wed. Thur. Fri. Sat. Sun.

BREAKFAST	Amount	Cal.	Fat gm	Carb. gm	Fiber gm	Sugar gm	Added sugar gm	Protein gm
🕐 TOTAL								

Insulin: Pre-sugar level: Post sugar level:

SNACK	Amount	Cal.	Fat gm	Carb. gm	Fiber gm	Sugar gm	Added sugar gm	Protein gm
🕐 TOTAL								

Insulin: Pre-sugar level: Post sugar level:

LUNCH	Amount	Cal.	Fat gm	Carb. gm	Fiber gm	Sugar gm	Added sugar gm	Protein gm
🕐 TOTAL								

Insulin: Pre-sugar level: Post sugar level:

SNACK	Amount	Cal.	Fat gm	Carb. gm	Fiber gm	Sugar gm	Added sugar gm	Protein gm
🕐 TOTAL								

Insulin: Pre-sugar level: Post sugar level:

8 oz

Step 2 – Tracking Food

DINNER	Amount	Cal.	Fat gm	Carb. gm	Fiber gm	Sugar gm	Added sugar gm	Protein gm
TOTAL								

Insulin: _____ Pre-sugar level: _____ Post sugar level: _____

SNACK	Amount	Cal.	Fat gm	Carb. gm	Fiber gm	Sugar gm	Added sugar gm	Protein gm
TOTAL								

Insulin: _____ Pre-sugar level: _____ Post sugar level: _____

| Daily Total | | | | | | | | |
| Daily Target | | | | | | | | |

Ketone Levels (mM)

0   0.5   1.0   1.5   2.0   2.5   3.0   5.0+

Exercise notes

What _____

Duration _____

Calories Burned _____

Vitamins / Supplements / Meds.

Description	Qty

How was today?

_____
_____
_____

DAILY

Date: Mon.   Tue.   Wed.   Thur.   Fri.   Sat.   Sun.

BREAKFAST	Amount	Cal.	Fat gm	Carb. gm	Fiber gm	Sugar gm	Added sugar gm	Protein gm
⊘ TOTAL								

Insulin: _____   Pre-sugar level: _____   Post sugar level: _____

SNACK	Amount	Cal.	Fat gm	Carb. gm	Fiber gm	Sugar gm	Added sugar gm	Protein gm
⊘ TOTAL								

Insulin: _____   Pre-sugar level: _____   Post sugar level: _____

LUNCH	Amount	Cal.	Fat gm	Carb. gm	Fiber gm	Sugar gm	Added sugar gm	Protein gm
⊘ TOTAL								

Insulin: _____   Pre-sugar level: _____   Post sugar level: _____

SNACK	Amount	Cal.	Fat gm	Carb. gm	Fiber gm	Sugar gm	Added sugar gm	Protein gm
⊘ TOTAL								

Insulin: _____   Pre-sugar level: _____   Post sugar level: _____

8 oz

Step 2 – Tracking Food

DINNER	Amount	Cal.	Fat gm	Carb. gm	Fiber gm	Sugar gm	Added sugar gm	Protein gm
ⓧ TOTAL								

Insulin: _____ Pre-sugar level: _____ Post sugar level: _____

SNACK	Amount	Cal.	Fat gm	Carb. gm	Fiber gm	Sugar gm	Added sugar gm	Protein gm
ⓧ TOTAL								

Insulin: _____ Pre-sugar level: _____ Post sugar level: _____

| Daily Total | | | | | | | | |
| Daily Target | | | | | | | | |

Ketone Levels (mM)

|—+—+—+—+—+—+—|
0   0.5 1.0 1.5 2.0 2.5 3.0   5.0+

Exercise notes

What _____

Duration _____

Calories Burned _____

Vitamins / Supplements / Meds.

Description	Qty

How was today?

_____

_____

DAILY

Date:　　　　　　　　　　　Mon.　Tue.　Wed.　Thur.　Fri.　Sat.　Sun.

BREAKFAST	Amount	Cal.	Fat gm	Carb. gm	Fiber gm	Sugar gm	Added sugar gm	Protein gm
TOTAL								

Insulin:　　　　Pre-sugar level:　　　　Post sugar level:

SNACK	Amount	Cal.	Fat gm	Carb. gm	Fiber gm	Sugar gm	Added sugar gm	Protein gm
TOTAL								

Insulin:　　　　Pre-sugar level:　　　　Post sugar level:

LUNCH	Amount	Cal.	Fat gm	Carb. gm	Fiber gm	Sugar gm	Added sugar gm	Protein gm
TOTAL								

Insulin:　　　　Pre-sugar level:　　　　Post sugar level:

SNACK	Amount	Cal.	Fat gm	Carb. gm	Fiber gm	Sugar gm	Added sugar gm	Protein gm
TOTAL								

Insulin:　　　　Pre-sugar level:　　　　Post sugar level:

        8 oz

Step 2 – Tracking Food

DINNER		Amount	Cal.	Fat gm	Carb. gm	Fiber gm	Sugar gm	Added sugar gm	Protein gm
	TOTAL								
Insulin:	Pre-sugar level:		Post sugar level:						

SNACK		Amount	Cal.	Fat gm	Carb. gm	Fiber gm	Sugar gm	Added sugar gm	Protein gm
	TOTAL								
Insulin:	Pre-sugar level:		Post sugar level:						
Daily Total									
Daily Target									

Ketone Levels (mM)

0   0.5   1.0   1.5   2.0   2.5   3.0   5.0+

Exercise notes

What _____

Duration _____

Calories Burned _____

Vitamins / Supplements / Meds.

Description	Qty

How was today?

_____

_____

DAILY

Date: _____ Mon. Tue. Wed. Thur. Fri. Sat. Sun.

BREAKFAST	Amount	Cal.	Fat gm	Carb. gm	Fiber gm	Sugar gm	Added sugar gm	Protein gm
🕐 TOTAL								

Insulin: _____ Pre-sugar level: _____ Post sugar level: _____

SNACK	Amount	Cal.	Fat gm	Carb. gm	Fiber gm	Sugar gm	Added sugar gm	Protein gm
🕐 TOTAL								

Insulin: _____ Pre-sugar level: _____ Post sugar level: _____

LUNCH	Amount	Cal.	Fat gm	Carb. gm	Fiber gm	Sugar gm	Added sugar gm	Protein gm
🕐 TOTAL								

Insulin: _____ Pre-sugar level: _____ Post sugar level: _____

SNACK	Amount	Cal.	Fat gm	Carb. gm	Fiber gm	Sugar gm	Added sugar gm	Protein gm
🕐 TOTAL								

Insulin: _____ Pre-sugar level: _____ Post sugar level: _____

8 oz

Step 2 – Tracking Food

DINNER		Amount	Cal.	Fat gm	Carb. gm	Fiber gm	Sugar gm	Added sugar gm	Protein gm
		TOTAL							
Insulin:	Pre-sugar level:			Post sugar level:					

SNACK		Amount	Cal.	Fat gm	Carb. gm	Fiber gm	Sugar gm	Added sugar gm	Protein gm
		TOTAL							
Insulin:	Pre-sugar level:			Post sugar level:					
Daily Total									
Daily Target									

Ketone Levels (mM)

|—+—+—+—+—+——|
0   0.5 1.0 1.5 2.0 2.5 3.0   5.0+

Exercise notes

What _____

Duration _____

Calories Burned _____

Vitamins / Supplements / Meds.

Description	Qty

How was today?

_____

_____

DAILY

Date: _____   Mon.   Tue.   Wed.   Thur.   Fri.   Sat.   Sun.

BREAKFAST	Amount	Cal.	Fat gm	Carb. gm	Fiber gm	Sugar gm	Added sugar gm	Protein gm
🕐 TOTAL								

Insulin: _____   Pre-sugar level: _____   Post sugar level: _____

SNACK	Amount	Cal.	Fat gm	Carb. gm	Fiber gm	Sugar gm	Added sugar gm	Protein gm
🕐 TOTAL								

Insulin: _____   Pre-sugar level: _____   Post sugar level: _____

LUNCH	Amount	Cal.	Fat gm	Carb. gm	Fiber gm	Sugar gm	Added sugar gm	Protein gm
🕐 TOTAL								

Insulin: _____   Pre-sugar level: _____   Post sugar level: _____

SNACK	Amount	Cal.	Fat gm	Carb. gm	Fiber gm	Sugar gm	Added sugar gm	Protein gm
🕐 TOTAL								

Insulin: _____   Pre-sugar level: _____   Post sugar level: _____

         8 oz

Step 2 – Tracking Food

DINNER		Amount	Cal.	Fat gm	Carb. gm	Fiber gm	Sugar gm	Added sugar gm	Protein gm
🕐	TOTAL								

Insulin: _____ Pre-sugar level: _____ Post sugar level: _____

SNACK		Amount	Cal.	Fat gm	Carb. gm	Fiber gm	Sugar gm	Added sugar gm	Protein gm
🕐	TOTAL								

Insulin: _____ Pre-sugar level: _____ Post sugar level: _____

Daily Total									
Daily Target									

Ketone Levels (mM)

|—|—|—|—|—|—|—|
0   0.5   1.0   1.5   2.0   2.5   3.0   5.0+

Exercise notes

What _____

Duration _____

Calories Burned _____

Vitamins / Supplements / Meds.

Description	Qty

How was today?

_____

_____

_____

DAILY

Date: _____ Mon. Tue. Wed. Thur. Fri. Sat. Sun.

BREAKFAST	Amount	Cal.	Fat gm	Carb. gm	Fiber gm	Sugar gm	Added sugar gm	Protein gm
🕐 TOTAL								

Insulin: _____ Pre-sugar level: _____ Post sugar level: _____

SNACK	Amount	Cal.	Fat gm	Carb. gm	Fiber gm	Sugar gm	Added sugar gm	Protein gm
🕐 TOTAL								

Insulin: _____ Pre-sugar level: _____ Post sugar level: _____

LUNCH	Amount	Cal.	Fat gm	Carb. gm	Fiber gm	Sugar gm	Added sugar gm	Protein gm
🕐 TOTAL								

Insulin: _____ Pre-sugar level: _____ Post sugar level: _____

SNACK	Amount	Cal.	Fat gm	Carb. gm	Fiber gm	Sugar gm	Added sugar gm	Protein gm
🕐 TOTAL								

Insulin: _____ Pre-sugar level: _____ Post sugar level: _____

         8 oz

Step 2 – Tracking Food

DINNER	Amount	Cal.	Fat gm	Carb. gm	Fiber gm	Sugar gm	Added sugar gm	Protein gm
TOTAL								

Insulin: _____ Pre-sugar level: _____ Post sugar level: _____

SNACK	Amount	Cal.	Fat gm	Carb. gm	Fiber gm	Sugar gm	Added sugar gm	Protein gm
TOTAL								

Insulin: _____ Pre-sugar level: _____ Post sugar level: _____

Daily Total								
Daily Target								

Ketone Levels (mM)

|—|—|—|—|—|—|—|
0 0.5 1.0 1.5 2.0 2.5 3.0   5.0+

Exercise notes

What _____

Duration _____

Calories Burned _____

Vitamins / Supplements / Meds.

Description	Qty

How was today?

_____

_____

_____

WEEKLY WINS

What went well this week? What can I take forward to next week?

Making next week even better

What have you learned this week? What could have been better?

_____
_____
_____
_____
_____

What can you implement next week to ensure success?

_____
_____
_____
_____
_____

Do not forget to record any measurements you wish to track weekly in the reference section.

> **"IF YOU KEEP GOOD FOOD IN YOUR FRIDGE, YOU WILL EAT GOODFOOD"**

WEEK OF ____

Date: Mon. Tue. Wed. Thur. Fri. Sat. Sun.

BREAKFAST	Amount	Cal.	Fat gm	Carb. gm	Fiber gm	Sugar gm	Added sugar gm	Protein gm
TOTAL								

Insulin: _____   Pre-sugar level: _____   Post sugar level: _____

SNACK	Amount	Cal.	Fat gm	Carb. gm	Fiber gm	Sugar gm	Added sugar gm	Protein gm
TOTAL								

Insulin: _____   Pre-sugar level: _____   Post sugar level: _____

LUNCH	Amount	Cal.	Fat gm	Carb. gm	Fiber gm	Sugar gm	Added sugar gm	Protein gm
TOTAL								

Insulin: _____   Pre-sugar level: _____   Post sugar level: _____

SNACK	Amount	Cal.	Fat gm	Carb. gm	Fiber gm	Sugar gm	Added sugar gm	Protein gm
TOTAL								

Insulin: _____   Pre-sugar level: _____   Post sugar level: _____

          8 oz

Step 2 – Tracking Food

DINNER	Amount	Cal.	Fat gm	Carb. gm	Fiber gm	Sugar gm	Added sugar gm	Protein gm
TOTAL								

Insulin: _____   Pre-sugar level: _____   Post sugar level: _____

SNACK	Amount	Cal.	Fat gm	Carb. gm	Fiber gm	Sugar gm	Added sugar gm	Protein gm
TOTAL								

Insulin: _____   Pre-sugar level: _____   Post sugar level: _____

| Daily Total | | | | | | | | |
| Daily Target | | | | | | | | |

Ketone Levels (mM)

0   0.5   1.0   1.5   2.0   2.5   3.0   5.0+

Vitamins / Supplements / Meds.

Description	Qty

Exercise notes

What _____

Duration _____

Calories Burned _____

How was today?

_____

_____

_____

DAILY

Date: Mon. Tue. Wed. Thur. Fri. Sat. Sun.

BREAKFAST	Amount	Cal.	Fat gm	Carb. gm	Fiber gm	Sugar gm	Added sugar gm	Protein gm
TOTAL								

Insulin: Pre-sugar level: Post sugar level:

SNACK	Amount	Cal.	Fat gm	Carb. gm	Fiber gm	Sugar gm	Added sugar gm	Protein gm
TOTAL								

Insulin: Pre-sugar level: Post sugar level:

LUNCH	Amount	Cal.	Fat gm	Carb. gm	Fiber gm	Sugar gm	Added sugar gm	Protein gm
TOTAL								

Insulin: Pre-sugar level: Post sugar level:

SNACK	Amount	Cal.	Fat gm	Carb. gm	Fiber gm	Sugar gm	Added sugar gm	Protein gm
TOTAL								

Insulin: Pre-sugar level: Post sugar level:

        8 oz

Step 2 – Tracking Food

DINNER	Amount	Cal.	Fat gm	Carb. gm	Fiber gm	Sugar gm	Added sugar gm	Protein gm
	TOTAL							

Insulin: Pre-sugar level: Post sugar level:

SNACK	Amount	Cal.	Fat gm	Carb. gm	Fiber gm	Sugar gm	Added sugar gm	Protein gm
	TOTAL							

Insulin: Pre-sugar level: Post sugar level:

| Daily Total | | | | | | | |
| Daily Target | | | | | | | |

Ketone Levels (mM)

0   0.5   1.0   1.5   2.0   2.5   3.0   5.0+

Exercise notes

What _____

Duration _____

Calories Burned _____

Vitamins / Supplements / Meds.

Description	Qty

How was today?

_____

_____

DAILY

Date: Mon. Tue. Wed. Thur. Fri. Sat. Sun.

BREAKFAST	Amount	Cal.	Fat gm	Carb. gm	Fiber gm	Sugar gm	Added sugar gm	Protein gm
TOTAL								

Insulin: Pre-sugar level: Post sugar level:

SNACK	Amount	Cal.	Fat gm	Carb. gm	Fiber gm	Sugar gm	Added sugar gm	Protein gm
TOTAL								

Insulin: Pre-sugar level: Post sugar level:

LUNCH	Amount	Cal.	Fat gm	Carb. gm	Fiber gm	Sugar gm	Added sugar gm	Protein gm
TOTAL								

Insulin: Pre-sugar level: Post sugar level:

SNACK	Amount	Cal.	Fat gm	Carb. gm	Fiber gm	Sugar gm	Added sugar gm	Protein gm
TOTAL								

Insulin: Pre-sugar level: Post sugar level:

8 oz

Step 2 – Tracking Food

DINNER	Amount	Cal.	Fat gm	Carb. gm	Fiber gm	Sugar gm	Added sugar gm	Protein gm
TOTAL								

Insulin: _____ Pre-sugar level: _____ Post sugar level: _____

SNACK	Amount	Cal.	Fat gm	Carb. gm	Fiber gm	Sugar gm	Added sugar gm	Protein gm
TOTAL								

Insulin: _____ Pre-sugar level: _____ Post sugar level: _____

| Daily Total | | | | | | | | |
| Daily Target | | | | | | | | |

Ketone Levels (mM)

0   0.5   1.0   1.5   2.0   2.5   3.0   5.0+

Exercise notes

What _____

Duration _____

Calories Burned _____

Vitamins / Supplements / Meds.

Description	Qty

How was today?

_____

_____

DAILY

Date: Mon.   Tue.   Wed.   Thur.   Fri.   Sat.   Sun.

BREAKFAST	Amount	Cal.	Fat gm	Carb. gm	Fiber gm	Sugar gm	Added sugar gm	Protein gm
TOTAL								

Insulin: _____   Pre-sugar level: _____   Post sugar level: _____

SNACK	Amount	Cal.	Fat gm	Carb. gm	Fiber gm	Sugar gm	Added sugar gm	Protein gm
TOTAL								

Insulin: _____   Pre-sugar level: _____   Post sugar level: _____

LUNCH	Amount	Cal.	Fat gm	Carb. gm	Fiber gm	Sugar gm	Added sugar gm	Protein gm
TOTAL								

Insulin: _____   Pre-sugar level: _____   Post sugar level: _____

SNACK	Amount	Cal.	Fat gm	Carb. gm	Fiber gm	Sugar gm	Added sugar gm	Protein gm
TOTAL								

Insulin: _____   Pre-sugar level: _____   Post sugar level: _____

        8 oz

Step 2 – Tracking Food

DINNER		Amount	Cal.	Fat gm	Carb. gm	Fiber gm	Sugar gm	Added sugar gm	Protein gm
🕐	TOTAL								

Insulin: _____ Pre-sugar level: _____ Post sugar level: _____

SNACK		Amount	Cal.	Fat gm	Carb. gm	Fiber gm	Sugar gm	Added sugar gm	Protein gm
🕐	TOTAL								

Insulin: _____ Pre-sugar level: _____ Post sugar level: _____

| Daily Total | | | | | | | | | |
| Daily Target | | | | | | | | | |

Ketone Levels (mM)

|—|—|—|—|—|—|—|
0   0.5   1.0   1.5   2.0   2.5   3.0   5.0+

Exercise notes

What _____

Duration _____

Calories Burned _____

Vitamins / Supplements / Meds.

Description	Qty

How was today?

_____

_____

DAILY

Date: Mon.   Tue.   Wed.   Thur.   Fri.   Sat.   Sun.

BREAKFAST	Amount	Cal.	Fat gm	Carb. gm	Fiber gm	Sugar gm	Added sugar gm	Protein gm
	TOTAL							

Insulin: Pre-sugar level: Post sugar level:

SNACK	Amount	Cal.	Fat gm	Carb. gm	Fiber gm	Sugar gm	Added sugar gm	Protein gm
	TOTAL							

Insulin: Pre-sugar level: Post sugar level:

LUNCH	Amount	Cal.	Fat gm	Carb. gm	Fiber gm	Sugar gm	Added sugar gm	Protein gm
	TOTAL							

Insulin: Pre-sugar level: Post sugar level:

SNACK	Amount	Cal.	Fat gm	Carb. gm	Fiber gm	Sugar gm	Added sugar gm	Protein gm
	TOTAL							

Insulin: Pre-sugar level: Post sugar level:

        8 oz

Step 2 – Tracking Food

DINNER	Amount	Cal.	Fat gm	Carb. gm	Fiber gm	Sugar gm	Added sugar gm	Protein gm
🕐 TOTAL								

Insulin: _____ Pre-sugar level: _____ Post sugar level: _____

SNACK	Amount	Cal.	Fat gm	Carb. gm	Fiber gm	Sugar gm	Added sugar gm	Protein gm
🕐 TOTAL								

Insulin: _____ Pre-sugar level: _____ Post sugar level: _____

| Daily Total | | | | | | | | |
| Daily Target | | | | | | | | |

Ketone Levels (mM)

0 — 0.5 — 1.0 — 1.5 — 2.0 — 2.5 — 3.0 — 5.0+

Exercise notes

What _____

Duration _____

Calories Burned _____

Vitamins / Supplements / Meds.

Description	Qty

How was today?

_____

_____

DAILY

Date: Mon.   Tue.   Wed.   Thur.   Fri.   Sat.   Sun.

BREAKFAST	Amount	Cal.	Fat gm	Carb. gm	Fiber gm	Sugar gm	Added sugar gm	Protein gm
	TOTAL							

Insulin: Pre-sugar level: Post sugar level:

SNACK	Amount	Cal.	Fat gm	Carb. gm	Fiber gm	Sugar gm	Added sugar gm	Protein gm
	TOTAL							

Insulin: Pre-sugar level: Post sugar level:

LUNCH	Amount	Cal.	Fat gm	Carb. gm	Fiber gm	Sugar gm	Added sugar gm	Protein gm
	TOTAL							

Insulin: Pre-sugar level: Post sugar level:

SNACK	Amount	Cal.	Fat gm	Carb. gm	Fiber gm	Sugar gm	Added sugar gm	Protein gm
	TOTAL							

Insulin: Pre-sugar level: Post sugar level:

8 oz

Step 2 – Tracking Food

DINNER	Amount	Cal.	Fat gm	Carb. gm	Fiber gm	Sugar gm	Added sugar gm	Protein gm
TOTAL								

Insulin: _____ Pre-sugar level: _____ Post sugar level: _____

SNACK	Amount	Cal.	Fat gm	Carb. gm	Fiber gm	Sugar gm	Added sugar gm	Protein gm
TOTAL								

Insulin: _____ Pre-sugar level: _____ Post sugar level: _____

| Daily Total | | | | | | | | |
| Daily Target | | | | | | | | |

Ketone Levels (mM)

|—|—|—|—|—|—|
0   0.5   1.0   1.5   2.0   2.5   3.0   5.0+

Exercise notes

What _____

Duration _____

Calories Burned _____

Vitamins / Supplements / Meds.

Description	Qty

How was today?

_____
_____
_____

DAILY

Date: _____   Mon. Tue. Wed. Thur. Fri. Sat. Sun.

BREAKFAST	Amount	Cal.	Fat gm	Carb. gm	Fiber gm	Sugar gm	Added sugar gm	Protein gm
🕐 TOTAL								

Insulin: _____   Pre-sugar level: _____   Post sugar level: _____

SNACK	Amount	Cal.	Fat gm	Carb. gm	Fiber gm	Sugar gm	Added sugar gm	Protein gm
🕐 TOTAL								

Insulin: _____   Pre-sugar level: _____   Post sugar level: _____

LUNCH	Amount	Cal.	Fat gm	Carb. gm	Fiber gm	Sugar gm	Added sugar gm	Protein gm
🕐 TOTAL								

Insulin: _____   Pre-sugar level: _____   Post sugar level: _____

SNACK	Amount	Cal.	Fat gm	Carb. gm	Fiber gm	Sugar gm	Added sugar gm	Protein gm
🕐 TOTAL								

Insulin: _____   Pre-sugar level: _____   Post sugar level: _____

         8 oz

Step 2 – Tracking Food

DINNER	Amount	Cal.	Fat gm	Carb. gm	Fiber gm	Sugar gm	Added sugar gm	Protein gm
TOTAL								

Insulin: _____ Pre-sugar level: _____ Post sugar level: _____

SNACK	Amount	Cal.	Fat gm	Carb. gm	Fiber gm	Sugar gm	Added sugar gm	Protein gm
TOTAL								

Insulin: _____ Pre-sugar level: _____ Post sugar level: _____

| Daily Total | | | | | | | | |
| Daily Target | | | | | | | | |

Ketone Levels (mM)

0   0.5   1.0   1.5   2.0   2.5   3.0   5.0+

Exercise notes

What _____

Duration _____

Calories Burned _____

Vitamins / Supplements / Meds.

Description	Qty

How was today?

_____

_____

WEEKLY WINS

What went well this week? What can I take forward to next week?

Making next week even better

What have you learned this week? What could have been better?

_____
_____
_____
_____
_____
_____

What can you implement next week to ensure success?

_____
_____
_____
_____
_____
_____

Do not forget to record any measurements you wish to track weekly in the reference section.

"FALL IN LOVE
WITH THE
PROCESS
AND THE
RESULTS
WILL COME"

WEEK OF ____

Date: Mon.   Tue.   Wed.   Thur.   Fri.   Sat.   Sun.

BREAKFAST	Amount	Cal.	Fat gm	Carb. gm	Fiber gm	Sugar gm	Added sugar gm	Protein gm
	TOTAL							

Insulin: _____ Pre-sugar level: _____ Post sugar level: _____

SNACK	Amount	Cal.	Fat gm	Carb. gm	Fiber gm	Sugar gm	Added sugar gm	Protein gm
	TOTAL							

Insulin: _____ Pre-sugar level: _____ Post sugar level: _____

LUNCH	Amount	Cal.	Fat gm	Carb. gm	Fiber gm	Sugar gm	Added sugar gm	Protein gm
	TOTAL							

Insulin: _____ Pre-sugar level: _____ Post sugar level: _____

SNACK	Amount	Cal.	Fat gm	Carb. gm	Fiber gm	Sugar gm	Added sugar gm	Protein gm
	TOTAL							

Insulin: _____ Pre-sugar level: _____ Post sugar level: _____

        8 oz

Step 2 – Tracking Food

DINNER	Amount	Cal.	Fat gm	Carb. gm	Fiber gm	Sugar gm	Added sugar gm	Protein gm
TOTAL								

Insulin: _____ Pre-sugar level: _____ Post sugar level: _____

SNACK	Amount	Cal.	Fat gm	Carb. gm	Fiber gm	Sugar gm	Added sugar gm	Protein gm
TOTAL								
Insulin: Pre-sugar level: Post sugar level:								
Daily Total								
Daily Target								

Ketone Levels (mM)

|—+—+—+—+—+—+—|
0   0.5   1.0   1.5   2.0   2.5   3.0   5.0+

Exercise notes

What _____

Duration _____

Calories Burned _____

Vitamins / Supplements / Meds.

Description	Qty

How was today?

_____

_____

_____

DAILY

Date: _____   Mon.   Tue.   Wed.   Thur.   Fri.   Sat.   Sun.

BREAKFAST	Amount	Cal.	Fat gm	Carb. gm	Fiber gm	Sugar gm	Added sugar gm	Protein gm
⏱ TOTAL								

Insulin: _____ Pre-sugar level: _____ Post sugar level: _____

SNACK	Amount	Cal.	Fat gm	Carb. gm	Fiber gm	Sugar gm	Added sugar gm	Protein gm
⏱ TOTAL								

Insulin: _____ Pre-sugar level: _____ Post sugar level: _____

LUNCH	Amount	Cal.	Fat gm	Carb. gm	Fiber gm	Sugar gm	Added sugar gm	Protein gm
⏱ TOTAL								

Insulin: _____ Pre-sugar level: _____ Post sugar level: _____

SNACK	Amount	Cal.	Fat gm	Carb. gm	Fiber gm	Sugar gm	Added sugar gm	Protein gm
⏱ TOTAL								

Insulin: _____ Pre-sugar level: _____ Post sugar level: _____

          8 oz

Step 2 – Tracking Food

DINNER	Amount	Cal.	Fat gm	Carb. gm	Fiber gm	Sugar gm	Added sugar gm	Protein gm
🕐 TOTAL								

Insulin: Pre-sugar level: Post sugar level:

SNACK	Amount	Cal.	Fat gm	Carb. gm	Fiber gm	Sugar gm	Added sugar gm	Protein gm
🕐 TOTAL								

Insulin: Pre-sugar level: Post sugar level:

Daily Total								
Daily Target								

Ketone Levels (mM)

0   0.5 1.0 1.5 2.0 2.5 3.0   5.0+

Exercise notes

What _____

Duration _____

Calories Burned _____

Vitamins / Supplements / Meds.

Description	Qty

How was today?

_____

_____

_____

DAILY

Date: Mon.   Tue.   Wed.   Thur.   Fri.   Sat.   Sun.

BREAKFAST	Amount	Cal.	Fat gm	Carb. gm	Fiber gm	Sugar gm	Added sugar gm	Protein gm
	TOTAL							

Insulin: Pre-sugar level: Post sugar level:

SNACK	Amount	Cal.	Fat gm	Carb. gm	Fiber gm	Sugar gm	Added sugar gm	Protein gm
	TOTAL							

Insulin: Pre-sugar level: Post sugar level:

LUNCH	Amount	Cal.	Fat gm	Carb. gm	Fiber gm	Sugar gm	Added sugar gm	Protein gm
	TOTAL							

Insulin: Pre-sugar level: Post sugar level:

SNACK	Amount	Cal.	Fat gm	Carb. gm	Fiber gm	Sugar gm	Added sugar gm	Protein gm
	TOTAL							

Insulin: Pre-sugar level: Post sugar level:

        8 oz

Step 2 – Tracking Food

DINNER	Amount	Cal.	Fat gm	Carb. gm	Fiber gm	Sugar gm	Added sugar gm	Protein gm
🕓 TOTAL								

Insulin: _____ Pre-sugar level: _____ Post sugar level: _____

SNACK	Amount	Cal.	Fat gm	Carb. gm	Fiber gm	Sugar gm	Added sugar gm	Protein gm
🕓 TOTAL								

Insulin: _____ Pre-sugar level: _____ Post sugar level: _____

| Daily Total | | | | | | | | |
| Daily Target | | | | | | | | |

Ketone Levels (mM)

|—|—|—|—|—|—|—|
0   0.5   1.0   1.5   2.0   2.5   3.0   5.0+

Exercise notes

What _____

Duration _____

Calories Burned _____

Vitamins / Supplements / Meds.

Description	Qty

How was today?

_____

_____

_____

DAILY

Date:　　　　　　　　　　　Mon.　Tue.　Wed.　Thur.　Fri.　Sat.　Sun.

BREAKFAST	Amount	Cal.	Fat gm	Carb. gm	Fiber gm	Sugar gm	Added sugar gm	Protein gm
TOTAL								

Insulin:　　　　Pre-sugar level:　　　　　Post sugar level:

SNACK	Amount	Cal.	Fat gm	Carb. gm	Fiber gm	Sugar gm	Added sugar gm	Protein gm
TOTAL								

Insulin:　　　　Pre-sugar level:　　　　　Post sugar level:

LUNCH	Amount	Cal.	Fat gm	Carb. gm	Fiber gm	Sugar gm	Added sugar gm	Protein gm
TOTAL								

Insulin:　　　　Pre-sugar level:　　　　　Post sugar level:

SNACK	Amount	Cal.	Fat gm	Carb. gm	Fiber gm	Sugar gm	Added sugar gm	Protein gm
TOTAL								

Insulin:　　　　Pre-sugar level:　　　　　Post sugar level:

8 oz

Step 2 – Tracking Food

DINNER	Amount	Cal.	Fat gm	Carb. gm	Fiber gm	Sugar gm	Added sugar gm	Protein gm
TOTAL								

Insulin: _____ Pre-sugar level: _____ Post sugar level: _____

SNACK	Amount	Cal.	Fat gm	Carb. gm	Fiber gm	Sugar gm	Added sugar gm	Protein gm
TOTAL								

Insulin: _____ Pre-sugar level: _____ Post sugar level: _____

| Daily Total | | | | | | | | |
| Daily Target | | | | | | | | |

Ketone Levels (mM)

0   0.5   1.0   1.5   2.0   2.5   3.0   5.0+

Exercise notes

What _____

Duration _____

Calories Burned _____

Vitamins / Supplements / Meds.

Description	Qty

How was today?

_____

_____

DAILY

Date: _____ Mon. Tue. Wed. Thur. Fri. Sat. Sun.

BREAKFAST	Amount	Cal.	Fat gm	Carb. gm	Fiber gm	Sugar gm	Added sugar gm	Protein gm
🕐 TOTAL								

Insulin: _____ Pre-sugar level: _____ Post sugar level: _____

SNACK	Amount	Cal.	Fat gm	Carb. gm	Fiber gm	Sugar gm	Added sugar gm	Protein gm
🕐 TOTAL								

Insulin: _____ Pre-sugar level: _____ Post sugar level: _____

LUNCH	Amount	Cal.	Fat gm	Carb. gm	Fiber gm	Sugar gm	Added sugar gm	Protein gm
🕐 TOTAL								

Insulin: _____ Pre-sugar level: _____ Post sugar level: _____

SNACK	Amount	Cal.	Fat gm	Carb. gm	Fiber gm	Sugar gm	Added sugar gm	Protein gm
🕐 TOTAL								

Insulin: _____ Pre-sugar level: _____ Post sugar level: _____

8 oz

Step 2 – Tracking Food

DINNER	Amount	Cal.	Fat gm	Carb. gm	Fiber gm	Sugar gm	Added sugar gm	Protein gm
⏱ TOTAL								

Insulin: _____ Pre-sugar level: _____ Post sugar level: _____

SNACK	Amount	Cal.	Fat gm	Carb. gm	Fiber gm	Sugar gm	Added sugar gm	Protein gm
⏱ TOTAL								

Insulin: _____ Pre-sugar level: _____ Post sugar level: _____

| Daily Total | | | | | | | | |
| Daily Target | | | | | | | | |

Ketone Levels (mM)

0   0.5   1.0   1.5   2.0   2.5   3.0   5.0+

Exercise notes

What _____

Duration _____

Calories Burned _____

Vitamins / Supplements / Meds.

Description	Qty

How was today?

_____

_____

DAILY

Date: Mon. Tue. Wed. Thur. Fri. Sat. Sun.

BREAKFAST	Amount	Cal.	Fat gm	Carb. gm	Fiber gm	Sugar gm	Added sugar gm	Protein gm
TOTAL								

Insulin: ____   Pre-sugar level: ____   Post sugar level: ____

SNACK	Amount	Cal.	Fat gm	Carb. gm	Fiber gm	Sugar gm	Added sugar gm	Protein gm
TOTAL								

Insulin: ____   Pre-sugar level: ____   Post sugar level: ____

LUNCH	Amount	Cal.	Fat gm	Carb. gm	Fiber gm	Sugar gm	Added sugar gm	Protein gm
TOTAL								

Insulin: ____   Pre-sugar level: ____   Post sugar level: ____

SNACK	Amount	Cal.	Fat gm	Carb. gm	Fiber gm	Sugar gm	Added sugar gm	Protein gm
TOTAL								

Insulin: ____   Pre-sugar level: ____   Post sugar level: ____

         8 oz

Step 2 – Tracking Food

DINNER	Amount	Cal.	Fat gm	Carb. gm	Fiber gm	Sugar gm	Added sugar gm	Protein gm
🕐 TOTAL								

Insulin: _____ Pre-sugar level: _____ Post sugar level: _____

SNACK	Amount	Cal.	Fat gm	Carb. gm	Fiber gm	Sugar gm	Added sugar gm	Protein gm
🕐 TOTAL								

Insulin: _____ Pre-sugar level: _____ Post sugar level: _____

| Daily Total | | | | | | | | |
| Daily Target | | | | | | | | |

Ketone Levels (mM)

|—|—|—|—|—|—|—|
0   0.5   1.0   1.5   2.0   2.5   3.0   5.0+

Exercise notes

What _____

Duration _____

Calories Burned _____

Vitamins / Supplements / Meds.	
Description	Qty

How was today?

_____

_____

DAILY

Date: _____   Mon. Tue. Wed. Thur. Fri. Sat. Sun.

BREAKFAST	Amount	Cal.	Fat gm	Carb. gm	Fiber gm	Sugar gm	Added sugar gm	Protein gm
🕒 TOTAL								

Insulin: _____   Pre-sugar level: _____   Post sugar level: _____

SNACK	Amount	Cal.	Fat gm	Carb. gm	Fiber gm	Sugar gm	Added sugar gm	Protein gm
🕒 TOTAL								

Insulin: _____   Pre-sugar level: _____   Post sugar level: _____

LUNCH	Amount	Cal.	Fat gm	Carb. gm	Fiber gm	Sugar gm	Added sugar gm	Protein gm
🕒 TOTAL								

Insulin: _____   Pre-sugar level: _____   Post sugar level: _____

SNACK	Amount	Cal.	Fat gm	Carb. gm	Fiber gm	Sugar gm	Added sugar gm	Protein gm
🕒 TOTAL								

Insulin: _____   Pre-sugar level: _____   Post sugar level: _____

8 oz

Step 2 – Tracking Food

DINNER	Amount	Cal.	Fat gm	Carb. gm	Fiber gm	Sugar gm	Added sugar gm	Protein gm
TOTAL								

Insulin: _____ Pre-sugar level: _____ Post sugar level: _____

SNACK	Amount	Cal.	Fat gm	Carb. gm	Fiber gm	Sugar gm	Added sugar gm	Protein gm
TOTAL								

Insulin: _____ Pre-sugar level: _____ Post sugar level: _____

| Daily Total | |
| Daily Target | |

Ketone Levels (mM)

0   0.5   1.0   1.5   2.0   2.5   3.0   5.0+

Exercise notes

What _____

Duration _____

Calories Burned _____

Vitamins / Supplements / Meds.

Description	Qty

How was today?

_____

_____

WEEKLY WINS

What went well this week? What can I take forward to next week?

Making next week even better

What have you learned this week? What could have been better?

_____
_____
_____
_____
_____
_____

What can you implement next week to ensure success?

_____
_____
_____
_____
_____
_____

Do not forget to record any measurements you wish to track weekly in the reference section.

> **"MOTIVATE THE MIND AND THE BODY WILL FOLLOW"**

WEEK OF ____

Date: _____   Mon. Tue. Wed. Thur. Fri. Sat. Sun.

BREAKFAST	Amount	Cal.	Fat gm	Carb. gm	Fiber gm	Sugar gm	Added sugar gm	Protein gm
🕒 TOTAL								

Insulin: _____ Pre-sugar level: _____ Post sugar level: _____

SNACK	Amount	Cal.	Fat gm	Carb. gm	Fiber gm	Sugar gm	Added sugar gm	Protein gm
🕒 TOTAL								

Insulin: _____ Pre-sugar level: _____ Post sugar level: _____

LUNCH	Amount	Cal.	Fat gm	Carb. gm	Fiber gm	Sugar gm	Added sugar gm	Protein gm
🕒 TOTAL								

Insulin: _____ Pre-sugar level: _____ Post sugar level: _____

SNACK	Amount	Cal.	Fat gm	Carb. gm	Fiber gm	Sugar gm	Added sugar gm	Protein gm
🕒 TOTAL								

Insulin: _____ Pre-sugar level: _____ Post sugar level: _____

         8 oz

Step 2 – Tracking Food

DINNER			Amount	Cal.	Fat gm	Carb. gm	Fiber gm	Sugar gm	Added sugar gm	Protein gm
🕐		TOTAL								
Insulin:	Pre-sugar level:			Post sugar level:						
SNACK			Amount	Cal.	Fat gm	Carb. gm	Fiber gm	Sugar gm	Added sugar gm	Protein gm
🕐		TOTAL								
Insulin:	Pre-sugar level:			Post sugar level:						
Daily Total										
Daily Target										

Ketone Levels (mM)

0   0.5   1.0   1.5   2.0   2.5   3.0   5.0+

Exercise notes

What _____

Duration _____

Calories Burned _____

Vitamins / Supplements / Meds.

Description	Qty

How was today?

_____

_____

DAILY

Date: Mon. Tue. Wed. Thur. Fri. Sat. Sun.

BREAKFAST	Amount	Cal.	Fat gm	Carb. gm	Fiber gm	Sugar gm	Added sugar gm	Protein gm
🕐 TOTAL								

Insulin: Pre-sugar level: Post sugar level:

SNACK	Amount	Cal.	Fat gm	Carb. gm	Fiber gm	Sugar gm	Added sugar gm	Protein gm
🕐 TOTAL								

Insulin: Pre-sugar level: Post sugar level:

LUNCH	Amount	Cal.	Fat gm	Carb. gm	Fiber gm	Sugar gm	Added sugar gm	Protein gm
🕐 TOTAL								

Insulin: Pre-sugar level: Post sugar level:

SNACK	Amount	Cal.	Fat gm	Carb. gm	Fiber gm	Sugar gm	Added sugar gm	Protein gm
🕐 TOTAL								

Insulin: Pre-sugar level: Post sugar level:

         8 oz

Step 2 – Tracking Food

DINNER	Amount	Cal.	Fat gm	Carb. gm	Fiber gm	Sugar gm	Added sugar gm	Protein gm
TOTAL								

Insulin: _____   Pre-sugar level: _____   Post sugar level: _____

SNACK	Amount	Cal.	Fat gm	Carb. gm	Fiber gm	Sugar gm	Added sugar gm	Protein gm
TOTAL								

Insulin: _____   Pre-sugar level: _____   Post sugar level: _____

| Daily Total | | | | | | | | |
| Daily Target | | | | | | | | |

Ketone Levels (mM)

0   0.5   1.0   1.5   2.0   2.5   3.0   5.0+

Exercise notes

What _____

Duration _____

Calories Burned _____

Vitamins / Supplements / Meds.

Description	Qty

How was today?

_____

_____

DAILY

Date: _____   Mon. Tue. Wed. Thur. Fri. Sat. Sun.

BREAKFAST	Amount	Cal.	Fat gm	Carb. gm	Fiber gm	Sugar gm	Added sugar gm	Protein gm
TOTAL								

Insulin: _____ Pre-sugar level: _____ Post sugar level: _____

SNACK	Amount	Cal.	Fat gm	Carb. gm	Fiber gm	Sugar gm	Added sugar gm	Protein gm
TOTAL								

Insulin: _____ Pre-sugar level: _____ Post sugar level: _____

LUNCH	Amount	Cal.	Fat gm	Carb. gm	Fiber gm	Sugar gm	Added sugar gm	Protein gm
TOTAL								

Insulin: _____ Pre-sugar level: _____ Post sugar level: _____

SNACK	Amount	Cal.	Fat gm	Carb. gm	Fiber gm	Sugar gm	Added sugar gm	Protein gm
TOTAL								

Insulin: _____ Pre-sugar level: _____ Post sugar level: _____

         8 oz

Step 2 – Tracking Food

DINNER	Amount	Cal.	Fat gm	Carb. gm	Fiber gm	Sugar gm	Added sugar gm	Protein gm
🕐 TOTAL								

Insulin: _____ Pre-sugar level: _____ Post sugar level: _____

SNACK	Amount	Cal.	Fat gm	Carb. gm	Fiber gm	Sugar gm	Added sugar gm	Protein gm
🕐 TOTAL								

Insulin: _____ Pre-sugar level: _____ Post sugar level: _____

| Daily Total | | | | | | | | |
| Daily Target | | | | | | | | |

Ketone Levels (mM)

| 0 | 0.5 | 1.0 | 1.5 | 2.0 | 2.5 | 3.0 | 5.0+ |

Exercise notes

What _____

Duration _____

Calories Burned _____

Vitamins / Supplements / Meds.

Description	Qty

How was today?

_____

_____

DAILY

Date: Mon. Tue. Wed. Thur. Fri. Sat. Sun.

BREAKFAST	Amount	Cal.	Fat gm	Carb. gm	Fiber gm	Sugar gm	Added sugar gm	Protein gm
TOTAL								

Insulin: Pre-sugar level: Post sugar level:

SNACK	Amount	Cal.	Fat gm	Carb. gm	Fiber gm	Sugar gm	Added sugar gm	Protein gm
TOTAL								

Insulin: Pre-sugar level: Post sugar level:

LUNCH	Amount	Cal.	Fat gm	Carb. gm	Fiber gm	Sugar gm	Added sugar gm	Protein gm
TOTAL								

Insulin: Pre-sugar level: Post sugar level:

SNACK	Amount	Cal.	Fat gm	Carb. gm	Fiber gm	Sugar gm	Added sugar gm	Protein gm
TOTAL								

Insulin: Pre-sugar level: Post sugar level:

        8 oz

Step 2 – Tracking Food

DINNER	Amount	Cal.	Fat gm	Carb. gm	Fiber gm	Sugar gm	Added sugar gm	Protein gm
🕐 TOTAL								

Insulin: _____ Pre-sugar level: _____ Post sugar level: _____

SNACK	Amount	Cal.	Fat gm	Carb. gm	Fiber gm	Sugar gm	Added sugar gm	Protein gm
🕐 TOTAL								

Insulin: _____ Pre-sugar level: _____ Post sugar level: _____

| Daily Total | | | | | | | | |
| Daily Target | | | | | | | | |

Ketone Levels (mM)

0   0.5   1.0   1.5   2.0   2.5   3.0   5.0+

Exercise notes

What _____

Duration _____

Calories Burned _____

Vitamins / Supplements / Meds.

Description	Qty

How was today?

_____

_____

_____

DAILY

Date: Mon.   Tue.   Wed.   Thur.   Fri.   Sat.   Sun.

BREAKFAST	Amount	Cal.	Fat gm	Carb. gm	Fiber gm	Sugar gm	Added sugar gm	Protein gm
TOTAL								

Insulin: Pre-sugar level: Post sugar level:

SNACK	Amount	Cal.	Fat gm	Carb. gm	Fiber gm	Sugar gm	Added sugar gm	Protein gm
TOTAL								

Insulin: Pre-sugar level: Post sugar level:

LUNCH	Amount	Cal.	Fat gm	Carb. gm	Fiber gm	Sugar gm	Added sugar gm	Protein gm
TOTAL								

Insulin: Pre-sugar level: Post sugar level:

SNACK	Amount	Cal.	Fat gm	Carb. gm	Fiber gm	Sugar gm	Added sugar gm	Protein gm
TOTAL								

Insulin: Pre-sugar level: Post sugar level:

8 oz

Step 2 – Tracking Food

DINNER	Amount	Cal.	Fat gm	Carb. gm	Fiber gm	Sugar gm	Added sugar gm	Protein gm
⏱ TOTAL								

Insulin: _____ Pre-sugar level: _____ Post sugar level: _____

SNACK	Amount	Cal.	Fat gm	Carb. gm	Fiber gm	Sugar gm	Added sugar gm	Protein gm
⏱ TOTAL								

Insulin: _____ Pre-sugar level: _____ Post sugar level: _____

| Daily Total | | | | | | | | |
| Daily Target | | | | | | | | |

Ketone Levels (mM)

|—|—|—|—|—|—|—|
0   0.5   1.0   1.5   2.0   2.5   3.0   5.0+

Exercise notes

What _____

Duration _____

Calories Burned _____

Vitamins / Supplements / Meds.

Description	Qty

How was today?

_____

_____

DAILY

Date: _____ Mon. Tue. Wed. Thur. Fri. Sat. Sun.

BREAKFAST	Amount	Cal.	Fat gm	Carb. gm	Fiber gm	Sugar gm	Added sugar gm	Protein gm
🕐 TOTAL								

Insulin: _____ Pre-sugar level: _____ Post sugar level: _____

SNACK	Amount	Cal.	Fat gm	Carb. gm	Fiber gm	Sugar gm	Added sugar gm	Protein gm
🕐 TOTAL								

Insulin: _____ Pre-sugar level: _____ Post sugar level: _____

LUNCH	Amount	Cal.	Fat gm	Carb. gm	Fiber gm	Sugar gm	Added sugar gm	Protein gm
🕐 TOTAL								

Insulin: _____ Pre-sugar level: _____ Post sugar level: _____

SNACK	Amount	Cal.	Fat gm	Carb. gm	Fiber gm	Sugar gm	Added sugar gm	Protein gm
🕐 TOTAL								

Insulin: _____ Pre-sugar level: _____ Post sugar level: _____

         8 oz

Step 2 – Tracking Food

DINNER	Amount	Cal.	Fat gm	Carb. gm	Fiber gm	Sugar gm	Added sugar gm	Protein gm
TOTAL								

Insulin: _____ Pre-sugar level: _____ Post sugar level: _____

SNACK	Amount	Cal.	Fat gm	Carb. gm	Fiber gm	Sugar gm	Added sugar gm	Protein gm
TOTAL								

Insulin: _____ Pre-sugar level: _____ Post sugar level: _____

| Daily Total | | | | | | | | |
| Daily Target | | | | | | | | |

Ketone Levels (mM)

| 0   0.5   1.0   1.5   2.0   2.5   3.0   5.0+ |

Exercise notes

What _____

Duration _____

Calories Burned _____

Vitamins / Supplements / Meds.

Description	Qty

How was today?

_____

_____

_____

DAILY

Date: Mon. Tue. Wed. Thur. Fri. Sat. Sun.

BREAKFAST	Amount	Cal.	Fat gm	Carb. gm	Fiber gm	Sugar gm	Added sugar gm	Protein gm
TOTAL								

Insulin: Pre-sugar level: Post sugar level:

SNACK	Amount	Cal.	Fat gm	Carb. gm	Fiber gm	Sugar gm	Added sugar gm	Protein gm
TOTAL								

Insulin: Pre-sugar level: Post sugar level:

LUNCH	Amount	Cal.	Fat gm	Carb. gm	Fiber gm	Sugar gm	Added sugar gm	Protein gm
TOTAL								

Insulin: Pre-sugar level: Post sugar level:

SNACK	Amount	Cal.	Fat gm	Carb. gm	Fiber gm	Sugar gm	Added sugar gm	Protein gm
TOTAL								

Insulin: Pre-sugar level: Post sugar level:

          8 oz

Step 2 – Tracking Food

DINNER	Amount	Cal.	Fat gm	Carb. gm	Fiber gm	Sugar gm	Added sugar gm	Protein gm
⏱ TOTAL								

Insulin: Pre-sugar level: Post sugar level:

SNACK	Amount	Cal.	Fat gm	Carb. gm	Fiber gm	Sugar gm	Added sugar gm	Protein gm
⏱ TOTAL								

Insulin: Pre-sugar level: Post sugar level:

| Daily Total | | | | | | | | |
| Daily Target | | | | | | | | |

Ketone Levels (mM)

0   0.5   1.0   1.5   2.0   2.5   3.0   5.0+

Exercise notes

What _____

Duration _____

Calories Burned _____

Vitamins / Supplements / Meds.

Description	Qty

How was today?

_____

_____

_____

WEEKLY WINS

What went well this week? What can I take forward to next week?

Making next week even better

What have you learned this week? What could have been better?

_____
_____
_____
_____
_____
_____

What can you implement next week to ensure success?

_____
_____
_____
_____
_____
_____

Do not forget to record any measurements you wish to track weekly in the reference section.

"YOU ARE WHAT YOU EAT. WHAT WOULD YOU LIKE TO BE TODAY?"

WEEK OF ____

Date:				Mon.	Tue.	Wed.	Thur.	Fri.	Sat.	Sun.
BREAKFAST	Amount	Cal.	Fat gm	Carb. gm	Fiber gm	Sugar gm	Added sugar gm	Protein gm		
🕐 _____ TOTAL										
Insulin: _____ Pre-sugar level: _____ Post sugar level: _____										

SNACK	Amount	Cal.	Fat gm	Carb. gm	Fiber gm	Sugar gm	Added sugar gm	Protein gm
🕐 _____ TOTAL								
Insulin: _____ Pre-sugar level: _____ Post sugar level: _____								

LUNCH	Amount	Cal.	Fat gm	Carb. gm	Fiber gm	Sugar gm	Added sugar gm	Protein gm
🕐 _____ TOTAL								
Insulin: _____ Pre-sugar level: _____ Post sugar level: _____								

SNACK	Amount	Cal.	Fat gm	Carb. gm	Fiber gm	Sugar gm	Added sugar gm	Protein gm
🕐 _____ TOTAL								
Insulin: _____ Pre-sugar level: _____ Post sugar level: _____								

        8 oz

Step 2 – Tracking Food

DINNER	Amount	Cal.	Fat gm	Carb. gm	Fiber gm	Sugar gm	Added sugar gm	Protein gm
TOTAL								

Insulin: ____ Pre-sugar level: ____ Post sugar level: ____

SNACK	Amount	Cal.	Fat gm	Carb. gm	Fiber gm	Sugar gm	Added sugar gm	Protein gm
TOTAL								

Insulin: ____ Pre-sugar level: ____ Post sugar level: ____

| Daily Total | | | | | | | |
| Daily Target | | | | | | | |

Ketone Levels (mM)

0   0.5   1.0   1.5   2.0   2.5   3.0   5.0+

Exercise notes

What _____

Duration _____

Calories Burned _____

Vitamins / Supplements / Meds.

Description	Qty

How was today?

_____

_____

_____

DAILY

Date: _____   Mon. Tue. Wed. Thur. Fri. Sat. Sun.

BREAKFAST	Amount	Cal.	Fat gm	Carb. gm	Fiber gm	Sugar gm	Added sugar gm	Protein gm
🕐 TOTAL								

Insulin: _____ Pre-sugar level: _____ Post sugar level: _____

SNACK	Amount	Cal.	Fat gm	Carb. gm	Fiber gm	Sugar gm	Added sugar gm	Protein gm
🕐 TOTAL								

Insulin: _____ Pre-sugar level: _____ Post sugar level: _____

LUNCH	Amount	Cal.	Fat gm	Carb. gm	Fiber gm	Sugar gm	Added sugar gm	Protein gm
🕐 TOTAL								

Insulin: _____ Pre-sugar level: _____ Post sugar level: _____

SNACK	Amount	Cal.	Fat gm	Carb. gm	Fiber gm	Sugar gm	Added sugar gm	Protein gm
🕐 TOTAL								

Insulin: _____ Pre-sugar level: _____ Post sugar level: _____

         8 oz

Step 2 – Tracking Food

DINNER		Amount	Cal.	Fat gm	Carb. gm	Fiber gm	Sugar gm	Added sugar gm	Protein gm
	TOTAL								
Insulin:	Pre-sugar level:		Post sugar level:						

SNACK		Amount	Cal.	Fat gm	Carb. gm	Fiber gm	Sugar gm	Added sugar gm	Protein gm
	TOTAL								
Insulin:	Pre-sugar level:		Post sugar level:						
Daily Total									
Daily Target									

Ketone Levels (mM)

0 0.5 1.0 1.5 2.0 2.5 3.0 5.0+

Exercise notes

What _____

Duration _____

Calories Burned _____

Vitamins / Supplements / Meds.

Description	Qty

How was today?

_____

_____

_____

DAILY

Date:	Mon. Tue. Wed. Thur. Fri. Sat. Sun.

BREAKFAST	Amount	Cal.	Fat gm	Carb. gm	Fiber gm	Sugar gm	Added sugar gm	Protein gm
TOTAL								

Insulin: ____ Pre-sugar level: ____ Post sugar level: ____

SNACK	Amount	Cal.	Fat gm	Carb. gm	Fiber gm	Sugar gm	Added sugar gm	Protein gm
TOTAL								

Insulin: ____ Pre-sugar level: ____ Post sugar level: ____

LUNCH	Amount	Cal.	Fat gm	Carb. gm	Fiber gm	Sugar gm	Added sugar gm	Protein gm
TOTAL								

Insulin: ____ Pre-sugar level: ____ Post sugar level: ____

SNACK	Amount	Cal.	Fat gm	Carb. gm	Fiber gm	Sugar gm	Added sugar gm	Protein gm
TOTAL								

Insulin: ____ Pre-sugar level: ____ Post sugar level: ____

8 oz

Step 2 – Tracking Food

DINNER	Amount	Cal.	Fat gm	Carb. gm	Fiber gm	Sugar gm	Added sugar gm	Protein gm
TOTAL								

Insulin: _____ Pre-sugar level: _____ Post sugar level: _____

SNACK	Amount	Cal.	Fat gm	Carb. gm	Fiber gm	Sugar gm	Added sugar gm	Protein gm
TOTAL								

Insulin: _____ Pre-sugar level: _____ Post sugar level: _____

| Daily Total | | | | | | | | |
| Daily Target | | | | | | | | |

Ketone Levels (mM)

0   0.5   1.0   1.5   2.0   2.5   3.0   5.0+

Exercise notes

What _____

Duration _____

Calories Burned _____

Vitamins / Supplements / Meds.

Description	Qty

How was today?

_____

_____

DAILY

Date: Mon. Tue. Wed. Thur. Fri. Sat. Sun.

BREAKFAST	Amount	Cal.	Fat gm	Carb. gm	Fiber gm	Sugar gm	Added sugar gm	Protein gm
🕐 TOTAL								

Insulin: Pre-sugar level: Post sugar level:

SNACK	Amount	Cal.	Fat gm	Carb. gm	Fiber gm	Sugar gm	Added sugar gm	Protein gm
🕐 TOTAL								

Insulin: Pre-sugar level: Post sugar level:

LUNCH	Amount	Cal.	Fat gm	Carb. gm	Fiber gm	Sugar gm	Added sugar gm	Protein gm
🕐 TOTAL								

Insulin: Pre-sugar level: Post sugar level:

SNACK	Amount	Cal.	Fat gm	Carb. gm	Fiber gm	Sugar gm	Added sugar gm	Protein gm
🕐 TOTAL								

Insulin: Pre-sugar level: Post sugar level:

8 oz

Step 2 – Tracking Food

DINNER	Amount	Cal.	Fat gm	Carb. gm	Fiber gm	Sugar gm	Added sugar gm	Protein gm
TOTAL								

Insulin: _____   Pre-sugar level: _____   Post sugar level: _____

SNACK	Amount	Cal.	Fat gm	Carb. gm	Fiber gm	Sugar gm	Added sugar gm	Protein gm
TOTAL								

Insulin: _____   Pre-sugar level: _____   Post sugar level: _____

| Daily Total | | | | | | | | |
| Daily Target | | | | | | | | |

Ketone Levels (mM)

|—|—|—|—|—|—|—|
0   0.5   1.0   1.5   2.0   2.5   3.0   5.0+

Exercise notes

What _____

Duration _____

Calories Burned _____

Vitamins / Supplements / Meds.

Description	Qty

How was today?

_____

_____

_____

DAILY

Date: Mon. Tue. Wed. Thur. Fri. Sat. Sun.

BREAKFAST	Amount	Cal.	Fat gm	Carb. gm	Fiber gm	Sugar gm	Added sugar gm	Protein gm
TOTAL								

Insulin: Pre-sugar level: Post sugar level:

SNACK	Amount	Cal.	Fat gm	Carb. gm	Fiber gm	Sugar gm	Added sugar gm	Protein gm
TOTAL								

Insulin: Pre-sugar level: Post sugar level:

LUNCH	Amount	Cal.	Fat gm	Carb. gm	Fiber gm	Sugar gm	Added sugar gm	Protein gm
TOTAL								

Insulin: Pre-sugar level: Post sugar level:

SNACK	Amount	Cal.	Fat gm	Carb. gm	Fiber gm	Sugar gm	Added sugar gm	Protein gm
TOTAL								

Insulin: Pre-sugar level: Post sugar level:

         8 oz

Step 2 – Tracking Food

DINNER	Amount	Cal.	Fat gm	Carb. gm	Fiber gm	Sugar gm	Added sugar gm	Protein gm
⏲ TOTAL								

Insulin: _____ Pre-sugar level: _____ Post sugar level: _____

SNACK	Amount	Cal.	Fat gm	Carb. gm	Fiber gm	Sugar gm	Added sugar gm	Protein gm
⏲ TOTAL								

Insulin: _____ Pre-sugar level: _____ Post sugar level: _____

Daily Total								
Daily Target								

Ketone Levels (mM)

0 0.5 1.0 1.5 2.0 2.5 3.0   5.0+

Exercise notes

What _____

Duration _____

Calories Burned _____

Vitamins / Supplements / Meds.

Description	Qty

How was today?

_____

_____

_____

DAILY

Date: Mon. Tue. Wed. Thur. Fri. Sat. Sun.

BREAKFAST	Amount	Cal.	Fat gm	Carb. gm	Fiber gm	Sugar gm	Added sugar gm	Protein gm
	TOTAL							

Insulin: Pre-sugar level: Post sugar level:

SNACK	Amount	Cal.	Fat gm	Carb. gm	Fiber gm	Sugar gm	Added sugar gm	Protein gm
	TOTAL							

Insulin: Pre-sugar level: Post sugar level:

LUNCH	Amount	Cal.	Fat gm	Carb. gm	Fiber gm	Sugar gm	Added sugar gm	Protein gm
	TOTAL							

Insulin: Pre-sugar level: Post sugar level:

SNACK	Amount	Cal.	Fat gm	Carb. gm	Fiber gm	Sugar gm	Added sugar gm	Protein gm
	TOTAL							

Insulin: Pre-sugar level: Post sugar level:

8 oz

Step 2 – Tracking Food

DINNER	Amount	Cal.	Fat gm	Carb. gm	Fiber gm	Sugar gm	Added sugar gm	Protein gm
TOTAL								

Insulin: _____   Pre-sugar level: _____   Post sugar level: _____

SNACK	Amount	Cal.	Fat gm	Carb. gm	Fiber gm	Sugar gm	Added sugar gm	Protein gm
TOTAL								

Insulin: _____   Pre-sugar level: _____   Post sugar level: _____

Daily Total							
Daily Target							

Ketone Levels (mM)

0   0.5   1.0   1.5   2.0   2.5   3.0   5.0+

Exercise notes

What _____

Duration _____

Calories Burned _____

Vitamins / Supplements / Meds.

Description	Qty

How was today?

_____

_____

DAILY

Date: _____   Mon. Tue. Wed. Thur. Fri. Sat. Sun.

BREAKFAST	Amount	Cal.	Fat gm	Carb. gm	Fiber gm	Sugar gm	Added sugar gm	Protein gm
🕐 TOTAL								

Insulin: _____ Pre-sugar level: _____ Post sugar level: _____

SNACK	Amount	Cal.	Fat gm	Carb. gm	Fiber gm	Sugar gm	Added sugar gm	Protein gm
🕐 TOTAL								

Insulin: _____ Pre-sugar level: _____ Post sugar level: _____

LUNCH	Amount	Cal.	Fat gm	Carb. gm	Fiber gm	Sugar gm	Added sugar gm	Protein gm
🕐 TOTAL								

Insulin: _____ Pre-sugar level: _____ Post sugar level: _____

SNACK	Amount	Cal.	Fat gm	Carb. gm	Fiber gm	Sugar gm	Added sugar gm	Protein gm
🕐 TOTAL								

Insulin: _____ Pre-sugar level: _____ Post sugar level: _____

8 oz

Step 2 – Tracking Food

DINNER	Amount	Cal.	Fat gm	Carb. gm	Fiber gm	Sugar gm	Added sugar gm	Protein gm
TOTAL								

Insulin: _____ Pre-sugar level: _____ Post sugar level: _____

SNACK	Amount	Cal.	Fat gm	Carb. gm	Fiber gm	Sugar gm	Added sugar gm	Protein gm
TOTAL								

Insulin: _____ Pre-sugar level: _____ Post sugar level: _____

| Daily Total | | | | | | | | |
| Daily Target | | | | | | | | |

Ketone Levels (mM)

0   0.5   1.0   1.5   2.0   2.5   3.0   5.0+

Exercise notes

What _____

Duration _____

Calories Burned _____

Vitamins / Supplements / Meds.

Description	Qty

How was today?

_____

_____

_____

WEEKLY WINS

What went well this week? What can I take forward to next week?

Making next week even better

What have you learned this week? What could have been better?

_____
_____
_____
_____
_____
_____

What can you implement next week to ensure success?

_____
_____
_____
_____
_____
_____

Do not forget to record any measurements you wish to track weekly in the reference section.

> **"YOUR LIFE DOES NOT GET BETTER BY CHANCE, IT GETS BETTER BY CHANGE"**

WEEK OF ____

Date:				Mon.	Tue.	Wed.	Thur.	Fri.	Sat.	Sun.
BREAKFAST		Amount	Cal.	Fat gm	Carb. gm	Fiber gm	Sugar gm	Added sugar gm	Protein gm
		TOTAL								
Insulin:	Pre-sugar level:		Post sugar level:							
SNACK		Amount	Cal.	Fat gm	Carb. gm	Fiber gm	Sugar gm	Added sugar gm	Protein gm
		TOTAL								
Insulin:	Pre-sugar level:		Post sugar level:							
LUNCH		Amount	Cal.	Fat gm	Carb. gm	Fiber gm	Sugar gm	Added sugar gm	Protein gm
		TOTAL								
Insulin:	Pre-sugar level:		Post sugar level:							
SNACK		Amount	Cal.	Fat gm	Carb. gm	Fiber gm	Sugar gm	Added sugar gm	Protein gm
		TOTAL								
Insulin:	Pre-sugar level:		Post sugar level:							

        8 oz

Step 2 – Tracking Food

DINNER	Amount	Cal.	Fat gm	Carb. gm	Fiber gm	Sugar gm	Added sugar gm	Protein gm
🕐 TOTAL								

Insulin: _____ Pre-sugar level: _____ Post sugar level: _____

SNACK	Amount	Cal.	Fat gm	Carb. gm	Fiber gm	Sugar gm	Added sugar gm	Protein gm
🕐 TOTAL								

Insulin: _____ Pre-sugar level: _____ Post sugar level: _____

| Daily Total | | | | | | | | |
| Daily Target | | | | | | | | |

Ketone Levels (mM)

0   0.5   1.0   1.5   2.0   2.5   3.0   5.0+

Vitamins / Supplements / Meds.

Description	Qty

Exercise notes

What _____

Duration _____

Calories Burned _____

How was today?

_____

_____

DAILY

Date: Mon.   Tue.   Wed.   Thur.   Fri.   Sat.   Sun.

BREAKFAST	Amount	Cal.	Fat gm	Carb. gm	Fiber gm	Sugar gm	Added sugar gm	Protein gm
TOTAL								

Insulin: Pre-sugar level: Post sugar level:

SNACK	Amount	Cal.	Fat gm	Carb. gm	Fiber gm	Sugar gm	Added sugar gm	Protein gm
TOTAL								

Insulin: Pre-sugar level: Post sugar level:

LUNCH	Amount	Cal.	Fat gm	Carb. gm	Fiber gm	Sugar gm	Added sugar gm	Protein gm
TOTAL								

Insulin: Pre-sugar level: Post sugar level:

SNACK	Amount	Cal.	Fat gm	Carb. gm	Fiber gm	Sugar gm	Added sugar gm	Protein gm
TOTAL								

Insulin: Pre-sugar level: Post sugar level:

        8 oz

Step 2 – Tracking Food

DINNER	Amount	Cal.	Fat gm	Carb. gm	Fiber gm	Sugar gm	Added sugar gm	Protein gm
TOTAL								

Insulin: _____ Pre-sugar level: _____ Post sugar level: _____

SNACK	Amount	Cal.	Fat gm	Carb. gm	Fiber gm	Sugar gm	Added sugar gm	Protein gm
TOTAL								

Insulin: _____ Pre-sugar level: _____ Post sugar level: _____

| Daily Total | | | | | | | | |
| Daily Target | | | | | | | | |

Ketone Levels (mM)

0   0.5   1.0   1.5   2.0   2.5   3.0   5.0+

Exercise notes

What _____

Duration _____

Calories Burned _____

Vitamins / Supplements / Meds.

Description	Qty

How was today?

_____

_____

_____

DAILY

Date: Mon. Tue. Wed. Thur. Fri. Sat. Sun.

BREAKFAST	Amount	Cal.	Fat gm	Carb. gm	Fiber gm	Sugar gm	Added sugar gm	Protein gm
⊙ TOTAL								

Insulin: Pre-sugar level: Post sugar level:

SNACK	Amount	Cal.	Fat gm	Carb. gm	Fiber gm	Sugar gm	Added sugar gm	Protein gm
⊙ TOTAL								

Insulin: Pre-sugar level: Post sugar level:

LUNCH	Amount	Cal.	Fat gm	Carb. gm	Fiber gm	Sugar gm	Added sugar gm	Protein gm
⊙ TOTAL								

Insulin: Pre-sugar level: Post sugar level:

SNACK	Amount	Cal.	Fat gm	Carb. gm	Fiber gm	Sugar gm	Added sugar gm	Protein gm
⊙ TOTAL								

Insulin: Pre-sugar level: Post sugar level:

          8 oz

Step 2 – Tracking Food

DINNER	Amount	Cal.	Fat gm	Carb. gm	Fiber gm	Sugar gm	Added sugar gm	Protein gm
⏱ TOTAL								

Insulin: _____ Pre-sugar level: _____ Post sugar level: _____

SNACK	Amount	Cal.	Fat gm	Carb. gm	Fiber gm	Sugar gm	Added sugar gm	Protein gm
⏱ TOTAL								

Insulin: _____ Pre-sugar level: _____ Post sugar level: _____

| Daily Total | | | | | | | | |
| Daily Target | | | | | | | | |

Ketone Levels (mM)

| 0   0.5   1.0   1.5   2.0   2.5   3.0   5.0+ |

Vitamins / Supplements / Meds.

Description	Qty

Exercise notes

What _____

Duration _____

Calories Burned _____

How was today?

_____

_____

_____

DAILY

Date:　　　　　　　　　　　Mon.　Tue.　Wed.　Thur.　Fri.　Sat.　Sun.

BREAKFAST	Amount	Cal.	Fat gm	Carb. gm	Fiber gm	Sugar gm	Added sugar gm	Protein gm
🕐 TOTAL								

Insulin: _____　Pre-sugar level: _____　Post sugar level: _____

SNACK	Amount	Cal.	Fat gm	Carb. gm	Fiber gm	Sugar gm	Added sugar gm	Protein gm
🕐 TOTAL								

Insulin: _____　Pre-sugar level: _____　Post sugar level: _____

LUNCH	Amount	Cal.	Fat gm	Carb. gm	Fiber gm	Sugar gm	Added sugar gm	Protein gm
🕐 TOTAL								

Insulin: _____　Pre-sugar level: _____　Post sugar level: _____

SNACK	Amount	Cal.	Fat gm	Carb. gm	Fiber gm	Sugar gm	Added sugar gm	Protein gm
🕐 TOTAL								

Insulin: _____　Pre-sugar level: _____　Post sugar level: _____

8 oz

Step 2 – Tracking Food

DINNER	Amount	Cal.	Fat gm	Carb. gm	Fiber gm	Sugar gm	Added sugar gm	Protein gm
TOTAL								

Insulin: _____ Pre-sugar level: _____ Post sugar level: _____

SNACK	Amount	Cal.	Fat gm	Carb. gm	Fiber gm	Sugar gm	Added sugar gm	Protein gm
TOTAL								

Insulin: _____ Pre-sugar level: _____ Post sugar level: _____

| Daily Total | | | | | | | | |
| Daily Target | | | | | | | | |

Ketone Levels (mM)

0   0.5   1.0   1.5   2.0   2.5   3.0   5.0+

Exercise notes

What _____

Duration _____

Calories Burned _____

Vitamins / Supplements / Meds.

Description	Qty

How was today?

_____

_____

_____

DAILY

Date: Mon. Tue. Wed. Thur. Fri. Sat. Sun.

BREAKFAST	Amount	Cal.	Fat gm	Carb. gm	Fiber gm	Sugar gm	Added sugar gm	Protein gm
⊘ TOTAL								

Insulin: ____ Pre-sugar level: ____ Post sugar level: ____

SNACK	Amount	Cal.	Fat gm	Carb. gm	Fiber gm	Sugar gm	Added sugar gm	Protein gm
⊘ TOTAL								

Insulin: ____ Pre-sugar level: ____ Post sugar level: ____

LUNCH	Amount	Cal.	Fat gm	Carb. gm	Fiber gm	Sugar gm	Added sugar gm	Protein gm
⊘ TOTAL								

Insulin: ____ Pre-sugar level: ____ Post sugar level: ____

SNACK	Amount	Cal.	Fat gm	Carb. gm	Fiber gm	Sugar gm	Added sugar gm	Protein gm
⊘ TOTAL								

Insulin: ____ Pre-sugar level: ____ Post sugar level: ____

        8 oz

Step 2 – Tracking Food

DINNER			Amount	Cal.	Fat gm	Carb. gm	Fiber gm	Sugar gm	Added sugar gm	Protein gm
🕒		TOTAL								
Insulin:	Pre-sugar level:			Post sugar level:						

SNACK			Amount	Cal.	Fat gm	Carb. gm	Fiber gm	Sugar gm	Added sugar gm	Protein gm
🕒		TOTAL								
Insulin:	Pre-sugar level:			Post sugar level:						
Daily Total										
Daily Target										

Ketone Levels (mM)

├──┼──┼──┼──┼──┼──┤
0   0.5 1.0 1.5 2.0 2.5 3.0   5.0+

Exercise notes

What _____

Duration _____

Calories Burned _____

Vitamins / Supplements / Meds.

Description	Qty

How was today?

_____

_____

_____

DAILY

Date: Mon. Tue. Wed. Thur. Fri. Sat. Sun.

BREAKFAST	Amount	Cal.	Fat gm	Carb. gm	Fiber gm	Sugar gm	Added sugar gm	Protein gm
	TOTAL							

Insulin: Pre-sugar level: Post sugar level:

SNACK	Amount	Cal.	Fat gm	Carb. gm	Fiber gm	Sugar gm	Added sugar gm	Protein gm
	TOTAL							

Insulin: Pre-sugar level: Post sugar level:

LUNCH	Amount	Cal.	Fat gm	Carb. gm	Fiber gm	Sugar gm	Added sugar gm	Protein gm
	TOTAL							

Insulin: Pre-sugar level: Post sugar level:

SNACK	Amount	Cal.	Fat gm	Carb. gm	Fiber gm	Sugar gm	Added sugar gm	Protein gm
	TOTAL							

Insulin: Pre-sugar level: Post sugar level:

8 oz

Step 2 – Tracking Food

DINNER	Amount	Cal.	Fat gm	Carb. gm	Fiber gm	Sugar gm	Added sugar gm	Protein gm
TOTAL								

Insulin: _____ Pre-sugar level: _____ Post sugar level: _____

SNACK	Amount	Cal.	Fat gm	Carb. gm	Fiber gm	Sugar gm	Added sugar gm	Protein gm
TOTAL								

Insulin: _____ Pre-sugar level: _____ Post sugar level: _____

| Daily Total | | | | | | | | |
| Daily Target | | | | | | | | |

Ketone Levels (mM)

0   0.5   1.0   1.5   2.0   2.5   3.0   5.0+

Exercise notes

What _____

Duration _____

Calories Burned _____

Vitamins / Supplements / Meds.

Description	Qty

How was today?

_____

_____

_____

DAILY

Date: _____ Mon. Tue. Wed. Thur. Fri. Sat. Sun.

BREAKFAST	Amount	Cal.	Fat gm	Carb. gm	Fiber gm	Sugar gm	Added sugar gm	Protein gm
🕐 TOTAL								

Insulin: _____ Pre-sugar level: _____ Post sugar level: _____

SNACK	Amount	Cal.	Fat gm	Carb. gm	Fiber gm	Sugar gm	Added sugar gm	Protein gm
🕐 TOTAL								

Insulin: _____ Pre-sugar level: _____ Post sugar level: _____

LUNCH	Amount	Cal.	Fat gm	Carb. gm	Fiber gm	Sugar gm	Added sugar gm	Protein gm
🕐 TOTAL								

Insulin: _____ Pre-sugar level: _____ Post sugar level: _____

SNACK	Amount	Cal.	Fat gm	Carb. gm	Fiber gm	Sugar gm	Added sugar gm	Protein gm
🕐 TOTAL								

Insulin: _____ Pre-sugar level: _____ Post sugar level: _____

8 oz

Step 2 – Tracking Food

DINNER	Amount	Cal.	Fat gm	Carb. gm	Fiber gm	Sugar gm	Added sugar gm	Protein gm
TOTAL								

Insulin: _____ Pre-sugar level: _____ Post sugar level: _____

SNACK	Amount	Cal.	Fat gm	Carb. gm	Fiber gm	Sugar gm	Added sugar gm	Protein gm
TOTAL								

Insulin: _____ Pre-sugar level: _____ Post sugar level: _____

| Daily Total | | | | | | | | |
| Daily Target | | | | | | | | |

Ketone Levels (mM)

|—|—|—|—|—|—|—|
0   0.5   1.0   1.5   2.0   2.5   3.0   5.0+

Exercise notes

What _____

Duration _____

Calories Burned _____

Vitamins / Supplements / Meds.

Description	Qty

How was today?

_____

_____

_____

WEEKLY WINS

What went well this week? What can I take forward to next week?

Making next week even better

What have you learned this week? What could have been better?

_____
_____
_____
_____
_____
_____

What can you implement next week to ensure success?

_____
_____
_____
_____
_____
_____

Do not forget to record any measurements you wish to track weekly in the reference section.

"THE GREATEST WEALTH IS YOUR HEALTH"

WEEK OF ____

Date:				Mon.	Tue.	Wed.	Thur.	Fri.	Sat.	Sun.
BREAKFAST			Amount	Cal.	Fat gm	Carb. gm	Fiber gm	Sugar gm	Added sugar gm	Protein gm
🕐		TOTAL								
Insulin:		Pre-sugar level:			Post sugar level:					
SNACK			Amount	Cal.	Fat gm	Carb. gm	Fiber gm	Sugar gm	Added sugar gm	Protein gm
🕐		TOTAL								
Insulin:		Pre-sugar level:			Post sugar level:					
LUNCH			Amount	Cal.	Fat gm	Carb. gm	Fiber gm	Sugar gm	Added sugar gm	Protein gm
🕐		TOTAL								
Insulin:		Pre-sugar level:			Post sugar level:					
SNACK			Amount	Cal.	Fat gm	Carb. gm	Fiber gm	Sugar gm	Added sugar gm	Protein gm
🕐		TOTAL								
Insulin:		Pre-sugar level:			Post sugar level:					

8 oz

Step 2 – Tracking Food

DINNER	Amount	Cal.	Fat gm	Carb. gm	Fiber gm	Sugar gm	Added sugar gm	Protein gm
🕐 TOTAL								

Insulin: _____ Pre-sugar level: _____ Post sugar level: _____

SNACK	Amount	Cal.	Fat gm	Carb. gm	Fiber gm	Sugar gm	Added sugar gm	Protein gm
🕐 TOTAL								

Insulin: _____ Pre-sugar level: _____ Post sugar level: _____

Daily Total								
Daily Target								

Ketone Levels (mM)

0 — 0.5 — 1.0 — 1.5 — 2.0 — 2.5 — 3.0 — 5.0+

Vitamins / Supplements / Meds.

Description	Qty

Exercise notes

What _____

Duration _____

Calories Burned _____

How was today?

_____

_____

_____

DAILY

Date: Mon.   Tue.   Wed.   Thur.   Fri.   Sat.   Sun.

BREAKFAST	Amount	Cal.	Fat gm	Carb. gm	Fiber gm	Sugar gm	Added sugar gm	Protein gm
TOTAL								

Insulin:_____ Pre-sugar level:_____ Post sugar level:_____

SNACK	Amount	Cal.	Fat gm	Carb. gm	Fiber gm	Sugar gm	Added sugar gm	Protein gm
TOTAL								

Insulin:_____ Pre-sugar level:_____ Post sugar level:_____

LUNCH	Amount	Cal.	Fat gm	Carb. gm	Fiber gm	Sugar gm	Added sugar gm	Protein gm
TOTAL								

Insulin:_____ Pre-sugar level:_____ Post sugar level:_____

SNACK	Amount	Cal.	Fat gm	Carb. gm	Fiber gm	Sugar gm	Added sugar gm	Protein gm
TOTAL								

Insulin:_____ Pre-sugar level:_____ Post sugar level:_____

8 oz

Step 2 – Tracking Food

DINNER	Amount	Cal.	Fat gm	Carb. gm	Fiber gm	Sugar gm	Added sugar gm	Protein gm
TOTAL								

Insulin: _____ Pre-sugar level: _____ Post sugar level: _____

SNACK	Amount	Cal.	Fat gm	Carb. gm	Fiber gm	Sugar gm	Added sugar gm	Protein gm
TOTAL								

Insulin: _____ Pre-sugar level: _____ Post sugar level: _____

| Daily Total | | | | | | | | |
| Daily Target | | | | | | | | |

Ketone Levels (mM)

0 — 0.5 — 1.0 — 1.5 — 2.0 — 2.5 — 3.0 — 5.0+

Exercise notes

What _____

Duration _____

Calories Burned _____

Vitamins / Supplements / Meds.

Description	Qty

How was today?

_____

_____

_____

DAILY

Date: Mon. Tue. Wed. Thur. Fri. Sat. Sun.

BREAKFAST	Amount	Cal.	Fat gm	Carb. gm	Fiber gm	Sugar gm	Added sugar gm	Protein gm
TOTAL								

Insulin: Pre-sugar level: Post sugar level:

SNACK	Amount	Cal.	Fat gm	Carb. gm	Fiber gm	Sugar gm	Added sugar gm	Protein gm
TOTAL								

Insulin: Pre-sugar level: Post sugar level:

LUNCH	Amount	Cal.	Fat gm	Carb. gm	Fiber gm	Sugar gm	Added sugar gm	Protein gm
TOTAL								

Insulin: Pre-sugar level: Post sugar level:

SNACK	Amount	Cal.	Fat gm	Carb. gm	Fiber gm	Sugar gm	Added sugar gm	Protein gm
TOTAL								

Insulin: Pre-sugar level: Post sugar level:

         8 oz

Step 2 – Tracking Food

DINNER	Amount	Cal.	Fat gm	Carb. gm	Fiber gm	Sugar gm	Added sugar gm	Protein gm
🕐 TOTAL								

Insulin: _____ Pre-sugar level: _____ Post sugar level: _____

SNACK	Amount	Cal.	Fat gm	Carb. gm	Fiber gm	Sugar gm	Added sugar gm	Protein gm
🕐 TOTAL								

Insulin: _____ Pre-sugar level: _____ Post sugar level: _____

| Daily Total | | | | | | | | |
| Daily Target | | | | | | | | |

Ketone Levels (mM)

0	0.5	1.0	1.5	2.0	2.5	3.0	5.0+

Exercise notes

What _____

Duration _____

Calories Burned _____

Vitamins / Supplements / Meds.

Description	Qty

How was today?

_____

_____

DAILY

Date: _____   Mon. Tue. Wed. Thur. Fri. Sat. Sun.

BREAKFAST	Amount	Cal.	Fat gm	Carb. gm	Fiber gm	Sugar gm	Added sugar gm	Protein gm
⏱ TOTAL								

Insulin: _____   Pre-sugar level: _____   Post sugar level: _____

SNACK	Amount	Cal.	Fat gm	Carb. gm	Fiber gm	Sugar gm	Added sugar gm	Protein gm
⏱ TOTAL								

Insulin: _____   Pre-sugar level: _____   Post sugar level: _____

LUNCH	Amount	Cal.	Fat gm	Carb. gm	Fiber gm	Sugar gm	Added sugar gm	Protein gm
⏱ TOTAL								

Insulin: _____   Pre-sugar level: _____   Post sugar level: _____

SNACK	Amount	Cal.	Fat gm	Carb. gm	Fiber gm	Sugar gm	Added sugar gm	Protein gm
⏱ TOTAL								

Insulin: _____   Pre-sugar level: _____   Post sugar level: _____

         8 oz

Step 2 – Tracking Food

DINNER	Amount	Cal.	Fat gm	Carb. gm	Fiber gm	Sugar gm	Added sugar gm	Protein gm
🕒 TOTAL								
Insulin:	Pre-sugar level:		Post sugar level:					

SNACK	Amount	Cal.	Fat gm	Carb. gm	Fiber gm	Sugar gm	Added sugar gm	Protein gm
🕒 TOTAL								
Insulin:	Pre-sugar level:		Post sugar level:					
Daily Total								
Daily Target								

Ketone Levels (mM)

|—+—+—+—+—+—+—|
0   0.5 1.0 1.5 2.0 2.5 3.0   5.0+

Exercise notes

What _____

Duration _____

Calories Burned _____

Vitamins / Supplements / Meds.

Description	Qty

How was today?

_____

_____

DAILY

Date: Mon. Tue. Wed. Thur. Fri. Sat. Sun.

BREAKFAST	Amount	Cal.	Fat gm	Carb. gm	Fiber gm	Sugar gm	Added sugar gm	Protein gm
	TOTAL							

Insulin: Pre-sugar level: Post sugar level:

SNACK	Amount	Cal.	Fat gm	Carb. gm	Fiber gm	Sugar gm	Added sugar gm	Protein gm
	TOTAL							

Insulin: Pre-sugar level: Post sugar level:

LUNCH	Amount	Cal.	Fat gm	Carb. gm	Fiber gm	Sugar gm	Added sugar gm	Protein gm
	TOTAL							

Insulin: Pre-sugar level: Post sugar level:

SNACK	Amount	Cal.	Fat gm	Carb. gm	Fiber gm	Sugar gm	Added sugar gm	Protein gm
	TOTAL							

Insulin: Pre-sugar level: Post sugar level:

8 oz

Step 2 – Tracking Food

DINNER	Amount	Cal.	Fat gm	Carb. gm	Fiber gm	Sugar gm	Added sugar gm	Protein gm
TOTAL								

Insulin: _____ Pre-sugar level: _____ Post sugar level: _____

SNACK	Amount	Cal.	Fat gm	Carb. gm	Fiber gm	Sugar gm	Added sugar gm	Protein gm
TOTAL								

Insulin: _____ Pre-sugar level: _____ Post sugar level: _____

| Daily Total | | | | | | | | |
| Daily Target | | | | | | | | |

Ketone Levels (mM)

0   0.5   1.0   1.5   2.0   2.5   3.0   5.0+

Exercise notes

What _____

Duration _____

Calories Burned _____

Vitamins / Supplements / Meds.

Description	Qty

How was today?

_____

_____

_____

DAILY

Date:　　　　　　　　　　Mon.　Tue.　Wed.　Thur.　Fri.　Sat.　Sun.

BREAKFAST	Amount	Cal.	Fat gm	Carb. gm	Fiber gm	Sugar gm	Added sugar gm	Protein gm
🕐 TOTAL								

Insulin:　　　　Pre-sugar level:　　　　Post sugar level:

SNACK	Amount	Cal.	Fat gm	Carb. gm	Fiber gm	Sugar gm	Added sugar gm	Protein gm
🕐 TOTAL								

Insulin:　　　　Pre-sugar level:　　　　Post sugar level:

LUNCH	Amount	Cal.	Fat gm	Carb. gm	Fiber gm	Sugar gm	Added sugar gm	Protein gm
🕐 TOTAL								

Insulin:　　　　Pre-sugar level:　　　　Post sugar level:

SNACK	Amount	Cal.	Fat gm	Carb. gm	Fiber gm	Sugar gm	Added sugar gm	Protein gm
🕐 TOTAL								

Insulin:　　　　Pre-sugar level:　　　　Post sugar level:

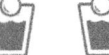   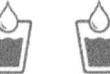   　8 oz

Step 2 – Tracking Food

DINNER	Amount	Cal.	Fat gm	Carb. gm	Fiber gm	Sugar gm	Added sugar gm	Protein gm
TOTAL								

Insulin: _____ Pre-sugar level: _____ Post sugar level: _____

SNACK	Amount	Cal.	Fat gm	Carb. gm	Fiber gm	Sugar gm	Added sugar gm	Protein gm
TOTAL								

Insulin: _____ Pre-sugar level: _____ Post sugar level: _____

| Daily Total | | | | | | | | |
| Daily Target | | | | | | | | |

Ketone Levels (mM)

0   0.5   1.0   1.5   2.0   2.5   3.0   5.0+

Exercise notes

What _____

Duration _____

Calories Burned _____

Vitamins / Supplements / Meds.

Description	Qty

How was today?

_____

_____

_____

DAILY

Date: Mon.   Tue.   Wed.   Thur.   Fri.   Sat.   Sun.

BREAKFAST	Amount	Cal.	Fat gm	Carb. gm	Fiber gm	Sugar gm	Added sugar gm	Protein gm
TOTAL								

Insulin: _____   Pre-sugar level: _____   Post sugar level: _____

SNACK	Amount	Cal.	Fat gm	Carb. gm	Fiber gm	Sugar gm	Added sugar gm	Protein gm
TOTAL								

Insulin: _____   Pre-sugar level: _____   Post sugar level: _____

LUNCH	Amount	Cal.	Fat gm	Carb. gm	Fiber gm	Sugar gm	Added sugar gm	Protein gm
TOTAL								

Insulin: _____   Pre-sugar level: _____   Post sugar level: _____

SNACK	Amount	Cal.	Fat gm	Carb. gm	Fiber gm	Sugar gm	Added sugar gm	Protein gm
TOTAL								

Insulin: _____   Pre-sugar level: _____   Post sugar level: _____

          8 oz

Step 2 – Tracking Food

DINNER	Amount	Cal.	Fat gm	Carb. gm	Fiber gm	Sugar gm	Added sugar gm	Protein gm
TOTAL								

Insulin: _____ Pre-sugar level: _____ Post sugar level: _____

SNACK	Amount	Cal.	Fat gm	Carb. gm	Fiber gm	Sugar gm	Added sugar gm	Protein gm
TOTAL								

Insulin: _____ Pre-sugar level: _____ Post sugar level: _____

Daily Total							
Daily Target							

Ketone Levels (mM)

|—|—|—|—|—|—|—|
0   0.5   1.0   1.5   2.0   2.5   3.0   5.0+

Exercise notes

What _____

Duration _____

Calories Burned _____

Vitamins / Supplements / Meds.

Description	Qty

How was today?

_____

_____

_____

WEEKLY WINS

What went well this week? What can I take forward to next week?

Making next week even better

What have you learned this week? What could have been better?

_____
_____
_____
_____
_____

What can you implement next week to ensure success?

_____
_____
_____
_____
_____
_____

Do not forget to record any measurements you wish to track weekly in the reference section.

> **"TODAY, I AM GOING TO TREAT YOU WELL. (NOTE TO SELF)"**

WEEK OF ____

Date:			Mon.	Tue.	Wed.	Thur.	Fri.	Sat.	Sun.
BREAKFAST	Amount	Cal.	Fat gm	Carb. gm	Fiber gm	Sugar gm	Added sugar gm	Protein gm	
		TOTAL							

Insulin: _____ Pre-sugar level: _____ Post sugar level: _____

SNACK	Amount	Cal.	Fat gm	Carb. gm	Fiber gm	Sugar gm	Added sugar gm	Protein gm
		TOTAL						

Insulin: _____ Pre-sugar level: _____ Post sugar level: _____

LUNCH	Amount	Cal.	Fat gm	Carb. gm	Fiber gm	Sugar gm	Added sugar gm	Protein gm
		TOTAL						

Insulin: _____ Pre-sugar level: _____ Post sugar level: _____

SNACK	Amount	Cal.	Fat gm	Carb. gm	Fiber gm	Sugar gm	Added sugar gm	Protein gm
		TOTAL						

Insulin: _____ Pre-sugar level: _____ Post sugar level: _____

        8 oz

Step 2 – Tracking Food

DINNER	Amount	Cal.	Fat gm	Carb. gm	Fiber gm	Sugar gm	Added sugar gm	Protein gm
⊙ TOTAL								

Insulin: _____   Pre-sugar level: _____   Post sugar level: _____

SNACK	Amount	Cal.	Fat gm	Carb. gm	Fiber gm	Sugar gm	Added sugar gm	Protein gm
⊙ TOTAL								

Insulin: _____   Pre-sugar level: _____   Post sugar level: _____

Daily Total								
Daily Target								

Ketone Levels (mM)

|—|—|—|—|—|—|—|
0   0.5   1.0   1.5   2.0   2.5   3.0   5.0+

Exercise notes

What _____

Duration _____

Calories Burned _____

Vitamins / Supplements / Meds.

Description	Qty

How was today?

_____

_____

_____

DAILY

Date: Mon. Tue. Wed. Thur. Fri. Sat. Sun.

BREAKFAST	Amount	Cal.	Fat gm	Carb. gm	Fiber gm	Sugar gm	Added sugar gm	Protein gm
TOTAL								

Insulin: Pre-sugar level: Post sugar level:

SNACK	Amount	Cal.	Fat gm	Carb. gm	Fiber gm	Sugar gm	Added sugar gm	Protein gm
TOTAL								

Insulin: Pre-sugar level: Post sugar level:

LUNCH	Amount	Cal.	Fat gm	Carb. gm	Fiber gm	Sugar gm	Added sugar gm	Protein gm
TOTAL								

Insulin: Pre-sugar level: Post sugar level:

SNACK	Amount	Cal.	Fat gm	Carb. gm	Fiber gm	Sugar gm	Added sugar gm	Protein gm
TOTAL								

Insulin: Pre-sugar level: Post sugar level:

         8 oz

Step 2 – Tracking Food

DINNER	Amount	Cal.	Fat gm	Carb. gm	Fiber gm	Sugar gm	Added sugar gm	Protein gm
🕒 TOTAL								

Insulin: _____ Pre-sugar level: _____ Post sugar level: _____

SNACK	Amount	Cal.	Fat gm	Carb. gm	Fiber gm	Sugar gm	Added sugar gm	Protein gm
🕒 TOTAL								

Insulin: _____ Pre-sugar level: _____ Post sugar level: _____

Daily Total							
Daily Target							

Ketone Levels (mM)

0   0.5   1.0   1.5   2.0   2.5   3.0   5.0+

Vitamins / Supplements / Meds.

Description	Qty

Exercise notes

What _____

Duration _____

Calories Burned _____

How was today?

_____

_____

_____

DAILY

Date: Mon. Tue. Wed. Thur. Fri. Sat. Sun.

BREAKFAST	Amount	Cal.	Fat gm	Carb. gm	Fiber gm	Sugar gm	Added sugar gm	Protein gm
TOTAL								

Insulin: _____ Pre-sugar level: _____ Post sugar level: _____

SNACK	Amount	Cal.	Fat gm	Carb. gm	Fiber gm	Sugar gm	Added sugar gm	Protein gm
TOTAL								

Insulin: _____ Pre-sugar level: _____ Post sugar level: _____

LUNCH	Amount	Cal.	Fat gm	Carb. gm	Fiber gm	Sugar gm	Added sugar gm	Protein gm
TOTAL								

Insulin: _____ Pre-sugar level: _____ Post sugar level: _____

SNACK	Amount	Cal.	Fat gm	Carb. gm	Fiber gm	Sugar gm	Added sugar gm	Protein gm
TOTAL								

Insulin: _____ Pre-sugar level: _____ Post sugar level: _____

8 oz

Step 2 – Tracking Food

DINNER	Amount	Cal.	Fat gm	Carb. gm	Fiber gm	Sugar gm	Added sugar gm	Protein gm
🕒 TOTAL								

Insulin: _____ Pre-sugar level: _____ Post sugar level: _____

SNACK	Amount	Cal.	Fat gm	Carb. gm	Fiber gm	Sugar gm	Added sugar gm	Protein gm
🕒 TOTAL								

Insulin: _____ Pre-sugar level: _____ Post sugar level: _____

| Daily Total | | | | | | | | |
| Daily Target | | | | | | | | |

Ketone Levels (mM)

|―――|―――|―――|―――|―――|―――|―――|
0   0.5   1.0   1.5   2.0   2.5   3.0   5.0+

Exercise notes

What _____

Duration _____

Calories Burned _____

Vitamins / Supplements / Meds.

Description	Qty

How was today?

_____

_____

DAILY

Date: Mon. Tue. Wed. Thur. Fri. Sat. Sun.

BREAKFAST	Amount	Cal.	Fat gm	Carb. gm	Fiber gm	Sugar gm	Added sugar gm	Protein gm
🕐 TOTAL								

Insulin: _____   Pre-sugar level: _____   Post sugar level: _____

SNACK	Amount	Cal.	Fat gm	Carb. gm	Fiber gm	Sugar gm	Added sugar gm	Protein gm
🕐 TOTAL								

Insulin: _____   Pre-sugar level: _____   Post sugar level: _____

LUNCH	Amount	Cal.	Fat gm	Carb. gm	Fiber gm	Sugar gm	Added sugar gm	Protein gm
🕐 TOTAL								

Insulin: _____   Pre-sugar level: _____   Post sugar level: _____

SNACK	Amount	Cal.	Fat gm	Carb. gm	Fiber gm	Sugar gm	Added sugar gm	Protein gm
🕐 TOTAL								

Insulin: _____   Pre-sugar level: _____   Post sugar level: _____

8 oz

Step 2 – Tracking Food

DINNER		Amount	Cal.	Fat gm	Carb. gm	Fiber gm	Sugar gm	Added sugar gm	Protein gm
🕒	TOTAL								
Insulin:	Pre-sugar level:		Post sugar level:						

SNACK		Amount	Cal.	Fat gm	Carb. gm	Fiber gm	Sugar gm	Added sugar gm	Protein gm
🕒	TOTAL								
Insulin:	Pre-sugar level:		Post sugar level:						
Daily Total									
Daily Target									

Ketone Levels (mM)

| 0 | 0.5 | 1.0 | 1.5 | 2.0 | 2.5 | 3.0 | 5.0+ |

Exercise notes

What _____

Duration _____

Calories Burned _____

Vitamins / Supplements / Meds.

Description	Qty

How was today?

_____

_____

DAILY

Date: _____   Mon. Tue. Wed. Thur. Fri. Sat. Sun.

BREAKFAST	Amount	Cal.	Fat gm	Carb. gm	Fiber gm	Sugar gm	Added sugar gm	Protein gm
🕐 TOTAL								

Insulin: _____ Pre-sugar level: _____ Post sugar level: _____

SNACK	Amount	Cal.	Fat gm	Carb. gm	Fiber gm	Sugar gm	Added sugar gm	Protein gm
🕐 TOTAL								

Insulin: _____ Pre-sugar level: _____ Post sugar level: _____

LUNCH	Amount	Cal.	Fat gm	Carb. gm	Fiber gm	Sugar gm	Added sugar gm	Protein gm
🕐 TOTAL								

Insulin: _____ Pre-sugar level: _____ Post sugar level: _____

SNACK	Amount	Cal.	Fat gm	Carb. gm	Fiber gm	Sugar gm	Added sugar gm	Protein gm
🕐 TOTAL								

Insulin: _____ Pre-sugar level: _____ Post sugar level: _____

         8 oz

Step 2 – Tracking Food

DINNER	Amount	Cal.	Fat gm	Carb. gm	Fiber gm	Sugar gm	Added sugar gm	Protein gm
⏱ TOTAL								

Insulin: _____ Pre-sugar level: _____ Post sugar level: _____

SNACK	Amount	Cal.	Fat gm	Carb. gm	Fiber gm	Sugar gm	Added sugar gm	Protein gm
⏱ TOTAL								

Insulin: _____ Pre-sugar level: _____ Post sugar level: _____

| Daily Total | | | | | | | | |
| Daily Target | | | | | | | | |

Ketone Levels (mM)

| 0 | 0.5 | 1.0 | 1.5 | 2.0 | 2.5 | 3.0 | 5.0+ |

Exercise notes

What _____

Duration _____

Calories Burned _____

Vitamins / Supplements / Meds.

Description	Qty

How was today?

_____

_____

DAILY

Date:　　　　　　　　　　Mon.　Tue.　Wed.　Thur.　Fri.　Sat.　Sun.

BREAKFAST	Amount	Cal.	Fat gm	Carb. gm	Fiber gm	Sugar gm	Added sugar gm	Protein gm
TOTAL								

Insulin:　　　　Pre-sugar level:　　　　Post sugar level:

SNACK	Amount	Cal.	Fat gm	Carb. gm	Fiber gm	Sugar gm	Added sugar gm	Protein gm
TOTAL								

Insulin:　　　　Pre-sugar level:　　　　Post sugar level:

LUNCH	Amount	Cal.	Fat gm	Carb. gm	Fiber gm	Sugar gm	Added sugar gm	Protein gm
TOTAL								

Insulin:　　　　Pre-sugar level:　　　　Post sugar level:

SNACK	Amount	Cal.	Fat gm	Carb. gm	Fiber gm	Sugar gm	Added sugar gm	Protein gm
TOTAL								

Insulin:　　　　Pre-sugar level:　　　　Post sugar level:

8 oz

Step 2 – Tracking Food

DINNER	Amount	Cal.	Fat gm	Carb. gm	Fiber gm	Sugar gm	Added sugar gm	Protein gm
TOTAL								

Insulin: _____ Pre-sugar level: _____ Post sugar level: _____

SNACK	Amount	Cal.	Fat gm	Carb. gm	Fiber gm	Sugar gm	Added sugar gm	Protein gm
TOTAL								

Insulin: _____ Pre-sugar level: _____ Post sugar level: _____

| Daily Total | | | | | | | | |
| Daily Target | | | | | | | | |

Ketone Levels (mM)

0   0.5   1.0   1.5   2.0   2.5   3.0   5.0+

Exercise notes

What _____

Duration _____

Calories Burned _____

Vitamins / Supplements / Meds.

Description	Qty

How was today?

_____

_____

DAILY

Date: Mon. Tue. Wed. Thur. Fri. Sat. Sun.

BREAKFAST	Amount	Cal.	Fat gm	Carb. gm	Fiber gm	Sugar gm	Added sugar gm	Protein gm
TOTAL								

Insulin: Pre-sugar level: Post sugar level:

SNACK	Amount	Cal.	Fat gm	Carb. gm	Fiber gm	Sugar gm	Added sugar gm	Protein gm
TOTAL								

Insulin: Pre-sugar level: Post sugar level:

LUNCH	Amount	Cal.	Fat gm	Carb. gm	Fiber gm	Sugar gm	Added sugar gm	Protein gm
TOTAL								

Insulin: Pre-sugar level: Post sugar level:

SNACK	Amount	Cal.	Fat gm	Carb. gm	Fiber gm	Sugar gm	Added sugar gm	Protein gm
TOTAL								

Insulin: Pre-sugar level: Post sugar level:

8 oz

Step 2 – Tracking Food

DINNER	Amount	Cal.	Fat gm	Carb. gm	Fiber gm	Sugar gm	Added sugar gm	Protein gm
TOTAL								

Insulin: _____ Pre-sugar level: _____ Post sugar level: _____

SNACK	Amount	Cal.	Fat gm	Carb. gm	Fiber gm	Sugar gm	Added sugar gm	Protein gm
TOTAL								

Insulin: _____ Pre-sugar level: _____ Post sugar level: _____

| Daily Total | | | | | | | | |
| Daily Target | | | | | | | | |

Ketone Levels (mM)

0 0.5 1.0 1.5 2.0 2.5 3.0 5.0+

Exercise notes

What _____

Duration _____

Calories Burned _____

Vitamins / Supplements / Meds.

Description	Qty

How was today?

_____

_____

_____

WEEKLY WINS

What went well this week? What can I take forward to next week?

Making next week even better

What have you learned this week? What could have been better?

_____
_____
_____
_____
_____
_____

What can you implement next week to ensure success?

_____
_____
_____
_____
_____
_____

Do not forget to record any measurements you wish to track weekly in the reference section.

> **"LIVE LESS OUT OF HABIT AND MORE OUT OF INTENT"**

WEEK OF _____

Date:				Mon.	Tue.	Wed.	Thur.	Fri.	Sat.	Sun.
BREAKFAST	Amount	Cal.	Fat gm	Carb. gm	Fiber gm	Sugar gm	Added sugar gm	Protein gm		
TOTAL										

Insulin: _____ Pre-sugar level: _____ Post sugar level: _____

SNACK	Amount	Cal.	Fat gm	Carb. gm	Fiber gm	Sugar gm	Added sugar gm	Protein gm
TOTAL								

Insulin: _____ Pre-sugar level: _____ Post sugar level: _____

LUNCH	Amount	Cal.	Fat gm	Carb. gm	Fiber gm	Sugar gm	Added sugar gm	Protein gm
TOTAL								

Insulin: _____ Pre-sugar level: _____ Post sugar level: _____

SNACK	Amount	Cal.	Fat gm	Carb. gm	Fiber gm	Sugar gm	Added sugar gm	Protein gm
TOTAL								

Insulin: _____ Pre-sugar level: _____ Post sugar level: _____

        8 oz

Step 2 – Tracking Food

DINNER	Amount	Cal.	Fat gm	Carb. gm	Fiber gm	Sugar gm	Added sugar gm	Protein gm
		TOTAL						

Insulin: _____ Pre-sugar level: _____ Post sugar level: _____

SNACK	Amount	Cal.	Fat gm	Carb. gm	Fiber gm	Sugar gm	Added sugar gm	Protein gm
		TOTAL						

Insulin: _____ Pre-sugar level: _____ Post sugar level: _____

| Daily Total | | | | | | | | |
| Daily Target | | | | | | | | |

Ketone Levels (mM)

0   0.5   1.0   1.5   2.0   2.5   3.0   5.0+

Exercise notes

What _____

Duration _____

Calories Burned _____

Vitamins / Supplements / Meds.

Description	Qty

How was today?

_____

_____

DAILY

Date: Mon. Tue. Wed. Thur. Fri. Sat. Sun.

BREAKFAST	Amount	Cal.	Fat gm	Carb. gm	Fiber gm	Sugar gm	Added sugar gm	Protein gm
	TOTAL							

Insulin: _____ Pre-sugar level: _____ Post sugar level: _____

SNACK	Amount	Cal.	Fat gm	Carb. gm	Fiber gm	Sugar gm	Added sugar gm	Protein gm
	TOTAL							

Insulin: _____ Pre-sugar level: _____ Post sugar level: _____

LUNCH	Amount	Cal.	Fat gm	Carb. gm	Fiber gm	Sugar gm	Added sugar gm	Protein gm
	TOTAL							

Insulin: _____ Pre-sugar level: _____ Post sugar level: _____

SNACK	Amount	Cal.	Fat gm	Carb. gm	Fiber gm	Sugar gm	Added sugar gm	Protein gm
	TOTAL							

Insulin: _____ Pre-sugar level: _____ Post sugar level: _____

8 oz

Step 2 – Tracking Food

DINNER	Amount	Cal.	Fat gm	Carb. gm	Fiber gm	Sugar gm	Added sugar gm	Protein gm
TOTAL								

Insulin: _____ Pre-sugar level: _____ Post sugar level: _____

SNACK	Amount	Cal.	Fat gm	Carb. gm	Fiber gm	Sugar gm	Added sugar gm	Protein gm
TOTAL								

Insulin: _____ Pre-sugar level: _____ Post sugar level: _____

| Daily Total | | | | | | | | |
| Daily Target | | | | | | | | |

Ketone Levels (mM)

| 0 | 0.5 | 1.0 | 1.5 | 2.0 | 2.5 | 3.0 | 5.0+ |

Exercise notes

What _____

Duration _____

Calories Burned _____

Vitamins / Supplements / Meds.

Description	Qty

How was today?

_____

_____

_____

DAILY

Date: Mon. Tue. Wed. Thur. Fri. Sat. Sun.

BREAKFAST	Amount	Cal.	Fat gm	Carb. gm	Fiber gm	Sugar gm	Added sugar gm	Protein gm
🕐 TOTAL								

Insulin: _____ Pre-sugar level: _____ Post sugar level: _____

SNACK	Amount	Cal.	Fat gm	Carb. gm	Fiber gm	Sugar gm	Added sugar gm	Protein gm
🕐 TOTAL								

Insulin: _____ Pre-sugar level: _____ Post sugar level: _____

LUNCH	Amount	Cal.	Fat gm	Carb. gm	Fiber gm	Sugar gm	Added sugar gm	Protein gm
🕐 TOTAL								

Insulin: _____ Pre-sugar level: _____ Post sugar level: _____

SNACK	Amount	Cal.	Fat gm	Carb. gm	Fiber gm	Sugar gm	Added sugar gm	Protein gm
🕐 TOTAL								

Insulin: _____ Pre-sugar level: _____ Post sugar level: _____

         8 oz

Step 2 – Tracking Food

DINNER	Amount	Cal.	Fat gm	Carb. gm	Fiber gm	Sugar gm	Added sugar gm	Protein gm
	TOTAL							

Insulin: _____ Pre-sugar level: _____ Post sugar level: _____

SNACK	Amount	Cal.	Fat gm	Carb. gm	Fiber gm	Sugar gm	Added sugar gm	Protein gm
	TOTAL							

Insulin: _____ Pre-sugar level: _____ Post sugar level: _____

| Daily Total | | | | | | | | |
| Daily Target | | | | | | | | |

Ketone Levels (mM)

0   0.5   1.0   1.5   2.0   2.5   3.0   5.0+

Exercise notes

What _____

Duration _____

Calories Burned _____

Vitamins / Supplements / Meds.

Description	Qty

How was today?

_____

_____

DAILY

Date: Mon.   Tue.   Wed.   Thur.   Fri.   Sat.   Sun.

BREAKFAST	Amount	Cal.	Fat gm	Carb. gm	Fiber gm	Sugar gm	Added sugar gm	Protein gm
TOTAL								

Insulin: _____   Pre-sugar level: _____   Post sugar level: _____

SNACK	Amount	Cal.	Fat gm	Carb. gm	Fiber gm	Sugar gm	Added sugar gm	Protein gm
TOTAL								

Insulin: _____   Pre-sugar level: _____   Post sugar level: _____

LUNCH	Amount	Cal.	Fat gm	Carb. gm	Fiber gm	Sugar gm	Added sugar gm	Protein gm
TOTAL								

Insulin: _____   Pre-sugar level: _____   Post sugar level: _____

SNACK	Amount	Cal.	Fat gm	Carb. gm	Fiber gm	Sugar gm	Added sugar gm	Protein gm
TOTAL								

Insulin: _____   Pre-sugar level: _____   Post sugar level: _____

8 oz

Step 2 – Tracking Food

DINNER	Amount	Cal.	Fat gm	Carb. gm	Fiber gm	Sugar gm	Added sugar gm	Protein gm
TOTAL								

Insulin: _____ Pre-sugar level: _____ Post sugar level: _____

SNACK	Amount	Cal.	Fat gm	Carb. gm	Fiber gm	Sugar gm	Added sugar gm	Protein gm
TOTAL								

Insulin: _____ Pre-sugar level: _____ Post sugar level: _____

| Daily Total | | | | | | | | |
| Daily Target | | | | | | | | |

Ketone Levels (mM)

0   0.5   1.0   1.5   2.0   2.5   3.0   5.0+

Exercise notes

What _____

Duration _____

Calories Burned _____

Vitamins / Supplements / Meds.

Description	Qty

How was today?

_____

_____

_____

DAILY

Date: _____   Mon. Tue. Wed. Thur. Fri. Sat. Sun.

BREAKFAST	Amount	Cal.	Fat gm	Carb. gm	Fiber gm	Sugar gm	Added sugar gm	Protein gm
	TOTAL							

Insulin: _____   Pre-sugar level: _____   Post sugar level: _____

SNACK	Amount	Cal.	Fat gm	Carb. gm	Fiber gm	Sugar gm	Added sugar gm	Protein gm
	TOTAL							

Insulin: _____   Pre-sugar level: _____   Post sugar level: _____

LUNCH	Amount	Cal.	Fat gm	Carb. gm	Fiber gm	Sugar gm	Added sugar gm	Protein gm
	TOTAL							

Insulin: _____   Pre-sugar level: _____   Post sugar level: _____

SNACK	Amount	Cal.	Fat gm	Carb. gm	Fiber gm	Sugar gm	Added sugar gm	Protein gm
	TOTAL							

Insulin: _____   Pre-sugar level: _____   Post sugar level: _____

         8 oz

Step 2 – Tracking Food

DINNER	Amount	Cal.	Fat gm	Carb. gm	Fiber gm	Sugar gm	Added sugar gm	Protein gm
🕐 TOTAL								

Insulin: ____ Pre-sugar level: ____ Post sugar level: ____

SNACK	Amount	Cal.	Fat gm	Carb. gm	Fiber gm	Sugar gm	Added sugar gm	Protein gm
🕐 TOTAL								

Insulin: ____ Pre-sugar level: ____ Post sugar level: ____

| Daily Total | | | | | | | | |
| Daily Target | | | | | | | | |

Ketone Levels (mM)

|—|—|—|—|—|—|—|
0   0.5   1.0   1.5   2.0   2.5   3.0   5.0+

Exercise notes

What _____

Duration _____

Calories Burned _____

Vitamins / Supplements / Meds.

Description	Qty

How was today?

_____

_____

_____

DAILY

Date:　　　　　　　　　　　Mon.　Tue.　Wed.　Thur.　Fri.　Sat.　Sun.

BREAKFAST	Amount	Cal.	Fat gm	Carb. gm	Fiber gm	Sugar gm	Added sugar gm	Protein gm
		TOTAL						

Insulin: _____　Pre-sugar level: _____　Post sugar level: _____

SNACK	Amount	Cal.	Fat gm	Carb. gm	Fiber gm	Sugar gm	Added sugar gm	Protein gm
		TOTAL						

Insulin: _____　Pre-sugar level: _____　Post sugar level: _____

LUNCH	Amount	Cal.	Fat gm	Carb. gm	Fiber gm	Sugar gm	Added sugar gm	Protein gm
		TOTAL						

Insulin: _____　Pre-sugar level: _____　Post sugar level: _____

SNACK	Amount	Cal.	Fat gm	Carb. gm	Fiber gm	Sugar gm	Added sugar gm	Protein gm
		TOTAL						

Insulin: _____　Pre-sugar level: _____　Post sugar level: _____

       　8 oz

Step 2 – Tracking Food

DINNER	Amount	Cal.	Fat gm	Carb. gm	Fiber gm	Sugar gm	Added sugar gm	Protein gm
🕐 TOTAL								

Insulin: _____ Pre-sugar level: _____ Post sugar level: _____

SNACK	Amount	Cal.	Fat gm	Carb. gm	Fiber gm	Sugar gm	Added sugar gm	Protein gm
🕐 TOTAL								

Insulin: _____ Pre-sugar level: _____ Post sugar level: _____

| Daily Total | | | | | | | | |
| Daily Target | | | | | | | | |

Ketone Levels (mM)

|—|—|—|—|—|—|—|
0   0.5 1.0 1.5 2.0 2.5 3.0   5.0+

Exercise notes

What _____

Duration _____

Calories Burned _____

Vitamins / Supplements / Meds.

Description	Qty

How was today?

_____

_____

_____

DAILY

Date: Mon. Tue. Wed. Thur. Fri. Sat. Sun.

BREAKFAST	Amount	Cal.	Fat gm	Carb. gm	Fiber gm	Sugar gm	Added sugar gm	Protein gm
TOTAL								

Insulin: Pre-sugar level: Post sugar level:

SNACK	Amount	Cal.	Fat gm	Carb. gm	Fiber gm	Sugar gm	Added sugar gm	Protein gm
TOTAL								

Insulin: Pre-sugar level: Post sugar level:

LUNCH	Amount	Cal.	Fat gm	Carb. gm	Fiber gm	Sugar gm	Added sugar gm	Protein gm
TOTAL								

Insulin: Pre-sugar level: Post sugar level:

SNACK	Amount	Cal.	Fat gm	Carb. gm	Fiber gm	Sugar gm	Added sugar gm	Protein gm
TOTAL								

Insulin: Pre-sugar level: Post sugar level:

8 oz

Step 2 – Tracking Food

DINNER	Amount	Cal.	Fat gm	Carb. gm	Fiber gm	Sugar gm	Added sugar gm	Protein gm
🕒 TOTAL								

Insulin: _____ Pre-sugar level: _____ Post sugar level: _____

SNACK	Amount	Cal.	Fat gm	Carb. gm	Fiber gm	Sugar gm	Added sugar gm	Protein gm
🕒 TOTAL								

Insulin: _____ Pre-sugar level: _____ Post sugar level: _____

| Daily Total | | | | | | | | |
| Daily Target | | | | | | | | |

Ketone Levels (mM)

|—+—+—+—+—+—+—|
0   0.5 1.0 1.5 2.0 2.5 3.0   5.0+

Exercise notes

What _____

Duration _____

Calories Burned _____

Vitamins / Supplements / Meds.

Description	Qty

How was today?

_____

_____

WEEKLY WINS

What went well this week? What can I take forward to next week?

Making next week even better

What have you learned this week? What could have been better?

_____
_____
_____
_____
_____
_____

What can you implement next week to ensure success?

_____
_____
_____
_____
_____
_____

Do not forget to record any measurements you wish to track weekly in the reference section.

> **"IT'S NOT ABOUT BEING THE BEST, IT'S ABOUT BEING SLIGHTLY BETTER THAN YOU WERE YESTERDAY"**

WEEK OF ____

Date: _____   Mon. Tue. Wed. Thur. Fri. Sat. Sun.

BREAKFAST	Amount	Cal.	Fat gm	Carb. gm	Fiber gm	Sugar gm	Added sugar gm	Protein gm
🕒 TOTAL								

Insulin: _____ Pre-sugar level: _____ Post sugar level: _____

SNACK	Amount	Cal.	Fat gm	Carb. gm	Fiber gm	Sugar gm	Added sugar gm	Protein gm
🕒 TOTAL								

Insulin: _____ Pre-sugar level: _____ Post sugar level: _____

LUNCH	Amount	Cal.	Fat gm	Carb. gm	Fiber gm	Sugar gm	Added sugar gm	Protein gm
🕒 TOTAL								

Insulin: _____ Pre-sugar level: _____ Post sugar level: _____

SNACK	Amount	Cal.	Fat gm	Carb. gm	Fiber gm	Sugar gm	Added sugar gm	Protein gm
🕒 TOTAL								

Insulin: _____ Pre-sugar level: _____ Post sugar level: _____

         8 oz

Step 2 – Tracking Food

DINNER	Amount	Cal.	Fat gm	Carb. gm	Fiber gm	Sugar gm	Added sugar gm	Protein gm
🕐 TOTAL								

Insulin: ____ Pre-sugar level: ____ Post sugar level: ____

SNACK	Amount	Cal.	Fat gm	Carb. gm	Fiber gm	Sugar gm	Added sugar gm	Protein gm
🕐 TOTAL								

Insulin: ____ Pre-sugar level: ____ Post sugar level: ____

Daily Total								
Daily Target								

Ketone Levels (mM)

|—|—|—|—|—|—|—|
0   0.5   1.0   1.5   2.0   2.5   3.0   5.0+

Exercise notes

What _____

Duration _____

Calories Burned _____

Vitamins / Supplements / Meds.

Description	Qty

How was today?

_____

_____

DAILY

Date: _____   Mon. Tue. Wed. Thur. Fri. Sat. Sun.

BREAKFAST	Amount	Cal.	Fat gm	Carb. gm	Fiber gm	Sugar gm	Added sugar gm	Protein gm
⏲ TOTAL								

Insulin: _____ Pre-sugar level: _____ Post sugar level: _____

SNACK	Amount	Cal.	Fat gm	Carb. gm	Fiber gm	Sugar gm	Added sugar gm	Protein gm
⏲ TOTAL								

Insulin: _____ Pre-sugar level: _____ Post sugar level: _____

LUNCH	Amount	Cal.	Fat gm	Carb. gm	Fiber gm	Sugar gm	Added sugar gm	Protein gm
⏲ TOTAL								

Insulin: _____ Pre-sugar level: _____ Post sugar level: _____

SNACK	Amount	Cal.	Fat gm	Carb. gm	Fiber gm	Sugar gm	Added sugar gm	Protein gm
⏲ TOTAL								

Insulin: _____ Pre-sugar level: _____ Post sugar level: _____

🥛 🥛 🥛 🥛 🥛 🥛 🥛 🥛   8 oz

Step 2 – Tracking Food

DINNER	Amount	Cal.	Fat gm	Carb. gm	Fiber gm	Sugar gm	Added sugar gm	Protein gm
TOTAL								

Insulin: _____   Pre-sugar level: _____   Post sugar level: _____

SNACK	Amount	Cal.	Fat gm	Carb. gm	Fiber gm	Sugar gm	Added sugar gm	Protein gm
TOTAL								

Insulin: _____   Pre-sugar level: _____   Post sugar level: _____

| Daily Total | | | | | | | | |
| Daily Target | | | | | | | | |

Ketone Levels (mM)

0   0.5   1.0   1.5   2.0   2.5   3.0   5.0+

Exercise notes

What _____

Duration _____

Calories Burned _____

Vitamins / Supplements / Meds.

Description	Qty

How was today?

_____

_____

DAILY

Date: _____ Mon. Tue. Wed. Thur. Fri. Sat. Sun.

BREAKFAST	Amount	Cal.	Fat gm	Carb. gm	Fiber gm	Sugar gm	Added sugar gm	Protein gm
TOTAL								

Insulin: _____ Pre-sugar level: _____ Post sugar level: _____

SNACK	Amount	Cal.	Fat gm	Carb. gm	Fiber gm	Sugar gm	Added sugar gm	Protein gm
TOTAL								

Insulin: _____ Pre-sugar level: _____ Post sugar level: _____

LUNCH	Amount	Cal.	Fat gm	Carb. gm	Fiber gm	Sugar gm	Added sugar gm	Protein gm
TOTAL								

Insulin: _____ Pre-sugar level: _____ Post sugar level: _____

SNACK	Amount	Cal.	Fat gm	Carb. gm	Fiber gm	Sugar gm	Added sugar gm	Protein gm
TOTAL								

Insulin: _____ Pre-sugar level: _____ Post sugar level: _____

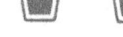 8 oz

Step 2 – Tracking Food

DINNER	Amount	Cal.	Fat gm	Carb. gm	Fiber gm	Sugar gm	Added sugar gm	Protein gm
🕐 TOTAL								

Insulin: _____ Pre-sugar level: _____ Post sugar level: _____

SNACK	Amount	Cal.	Fat gm	Carb. gm	Fiber gm	Sugar gm	Added sugar gm	Protein gm
🕐 TOTAL								

Insulin: _____ Pre-sugar level: _____ Post sugar level: _____

| Daily Total | | | | | | | | |
| Daily Target | | | | | | | | |

Ketone Levels (mM)

|—|—|—|—|—|—|—|
0   0.5   1.0   1.5   2.0   2.5   3.0   5.0+

Exercise notes

What _____

Duration _____

Calories Burned _____

Vitamins / Supplements / Meds.

Description	Qty

How was today?

_____

_____

_____

DAILY

Date: _____ Mon. Tue. Wed. Thur. Fri. Sat. Sun.

BREAKFAST	Amount	Cal.	Fat gm	Carb. gm	Fiber gm	Sugar gm	Added sugar gm	Protein gm
TOTAL								

Insulin: _____ Pre-sugar level: _____ Post sugar level: _____

SNACK	Amount	Cal.	Fat gm	Carb. gm	Fiber gm	Sugar gm	Added sugar gm	Protein gm
TOTAL								

Insulin: _____ Pre-sugar level: _____ Post sugar level: _____

LUNCH	Amount	Cal.	Fat gm	Carb. gm	Fiber gm	Sugar gm	Added sugar gm	Protein gm
TOTAL								

Insulin: _____ Pre-sugar level: _____ Post sugar level: _____

SNACK	Amount	Cal.	Fat gm	Carb. gm	Fiber gm	Sugar gm	Added sugar gm	Protein gm
TOTAL								

Insulin: _____ Pre-sugar level: _____ Post sugar level: _____

        8 oz

Step 2 – Tracking Food

DINNER	Amount	Cal.	Fat gm	Carb. gm	Fiber gm	Sugar gm	Added sugar gm	Protein gm
🕓 TOTAL								

Insulin: _____ Pre-sugar level: _____ Post sugar level: _____

SNACK	Amount	Cal.	Fat gm	Carb. gm	Fiber gm	Sugar gm	Added sugar gm	Protein gm
🕓 TOTAL								

Insulin: _____ Pre-sugar level: _____ Post sugar level: _____

| Daily Total | | | | | | | | |
| Daily Target | | | | | | | | |

Ketone Levels (mM)

|—|—|—|—|—|—|—|
0   0.5   1.0   1.5   2.0   2.5   3.0   5.0+

Exercise notes

What _____

Duration _____

Calories Burned _____

Vitamins / Supplements / Meds.

Description	Qty

How was today?

_____

_____

_____

DAILY

Date: _____ Mon. Tue. Wed. Thur. Fri. Sat. Sun.

BREAKFAST	Amount	Cal.	Fat gm	Carb. gm	Fiber gm	Sugar gm	Added sugar gm	Protein gm
⏲ TOTAL								

Insulin: _____ Pre-sugar level: _____ Post sugar level: _____

SNACK	Amount	Cal.	Fat gm	Carb. gm	Fiber gm	Sugar gm	Added sugar gm	Protein gm
⏲ TOTAL								

Insulin: _____ Pre-sugar level: _____ Post sugar level: _____

LUNCH	Amount	Cal.	Fat gm	Carb. gm	Fiber gm	Sugar gm	Added sugar gm	Protein gm
⏲ TOTAL								

Insulin: _____ Pre-sugar level: _____ Post sugar level: _____

SNACK	Amount	Cal.	Fat gm	Carb. gm	Fiber gm	Sugar gm	Added sugar gm	Protein gm
⏲ TOTAL								

Insulin: _____ Pre-sugar level: _____ Post sugar level: _____

8 oz

Step 2 – Tracking Food

DINNER	Amount	Cal.	Fat gm	Carb. gm	Fiber gm	Sugar gm	Added sugar gm	Protein gm
TOTAL								

Insulin: _____ Pre-sugar level: _____ Post sugar level: _____

SNACK	Amount	Cal.	Fat gm	Carb. gm	Fiber gm	Sugar gm	Added sugar gm	Protein gm
TOTAL								

Insulin: _____ Pre-sugar level: _____ Post sugar level: _____

| Daily Total | | | | | | | | |
| Daily Target | | | | | | | | |

Ketone Levels (mM)

├─┼─┼─┼─┼─┼─┤
0   0.5   1.0   1.5   2.0   2.5   3.0   5.0+

Exercise notes

What _____

Duration _____

Calories Burned _____

Vitamins / Supplements / Meds.

Description	Qty

How was today?

_____

_____

_____

DAILY

Date: _____   Mon.   Tue.   Wed.   Thur.   Fri.   Sat.   Sun.

BREAKFAST	Amount	Cal.	Fat gm	Carb. gm	Fiber gm	Sugar gm	Added sugar gm	Protein gm
TOTAL								

Insulin: _____ Pre-sugar level: _____ Post sugar level: _____

SNACK	Amount	Cal.	Fat gm	Carb. gm	Fiber gm	Sugar gm	Added sugar gm	Protein gm
TOTAL								

Insulin: _____ Pre-sugar level: _____ Post sugar level: _____

LUNCH	Amount	Cal.	Fat gm	Carb. gm	Fiber gm	Sugar gm	Added sugar gm	Protein gm
TOTAL								

Insulin: _____ Pre-sugar level: _____ Post sugar level: _____

SNACK	Amount	Cal.	Fat gm	Carb. gm	Fiber gm	Sugar gm	Added sugar gm	Protein gm
TOTAL								

Insulin: _____ Pre-sugar level: _____ Post sugar level: _____

          8 oz

Step 2 – Tracking Food

DINNER		Amount	Cal.	Fat gm	Carb. gm	Fiber gm	Sugar gm	Added sugar gm	Protein gm
⊙	TOTAL								

Insulin: _____ Pre-sugar level: _____ Post sugar level: _____

SNACK		Amount	Cal.	Fat gm	Carb. gm	Fiber gm	Sugar gm	Added sugar gm	Protein gm
⊙	TOTAL								

Insulin: _____ Pre-sugar level: _____ Post sugar level: _____

| Daily Total | | | | | | | | |
| Daily Target | | | | | | | | |

Ketone Levels (mM)

|—|—|—|—|—|—|—|
0   0.5 1.0 1.5 2.0 2.5 3.0   5.0+

Exercise notes

What _____

Duration _____

Calories Burned _____

Vitamins / Supplements / Meds.

Description	Qty

How was today?

_____

_____

_____

DAILY

Date: _____   Mon.   Tue.   Wed.   Thur.   Fri.   Sat.   Sun.

BREAKFAST	Amount	Cal.	Fat gm	Carb. gm	Fiber gm	Sugar gm	Added sugar gm	Protein gm
	TOTAL							

Insulin: _____   Pre-sugar level: _____   Post sugar level: _____

SNACK	Amount	Cal.	Fat gm	Carb. gm	Fiber gm	Sugar gm	Added sugar gm	Protein gm
	TOTAL							

Insulin: _____   Pre-sugar level: _____   Post sugar level: _____

LUNCH	Amount	Cal.	Fat gm	Carb. gm	Fiber gm	Sugar gm	Added sugar gm	Protein gm
	TOTAL							

Insulin: _____   Pre-sugar level: _____   Post sugar level: _____

SNACK	Amount	Cal.	Fat gm	Carb. gm	Fiber gm	Sugar gm	Added sugar gm	Protein gm
	TOTAL							

Insulin: _____   Pre-sugar level: _____   Post sugar level: _____

          8 oz

Step 2 – Tracking Food

DINNER	Amount	Cal.	Fat gm	Carb. gm	Fiber gm	Sugar gm	Added sugar gm	Protein gm
🕒 TOTAL								

Insulin: _____ Pre-sugar level: _____ Post sugar level: _____

SNACK	Amount	Cal.	Fat gm	Carb. gm	Fiber gm	Sugar gm	Added sugar gm	Protein gm
🕒 TOTAL								

Insulin: _____ Pre-sugar level: _____ Post sugar level: _____

| Daily Total | | | | | | | | |
| Daily Target | | | | | | | | |

Ketone Levels (mM)

|—|—|—|—|—|—|—|
0   0.5   1.0   1.5   2.0   2.5   3.0   5.0+

Exercise notes

What _____

Duration _____

Calories Burned _____

Vitamins / Supplements / Meds.

Description	Qty

How was today?

_____

_____

_____

> **"IT'S NOT A SHORT TERM DIET, IT'S A LONG TERM LIFESTYLE CHANGE"**

STEP 3
REVIEW

Reviewing your progress keeps you motivated. It shows how far you have come and encourages you to keep going when it gets hard.

In this section you can record your vital statistics across time as well as before and after measurements.

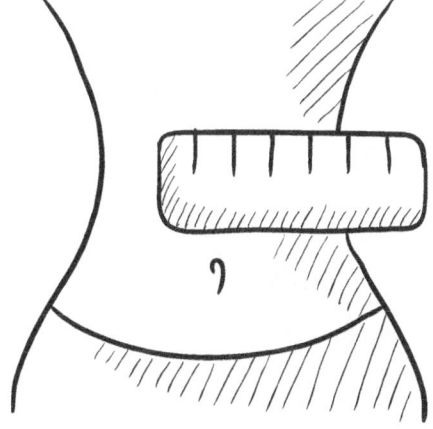

BEFORE AND AFTER

Record your before-and-after statistics to see how far you have come. Record as many or as few as you like.

Set the date for the before and after. We'd recommend three months from now, which is one cycle of the journal.

There are blank rows if you want to track anything specific.Tips:

	BEFORE	AFTER	CHANGE	GOAL
Date	Jan. 1st	Mar. 30th		
Weight	180lbs	160lbs	-20lbs	165lbs
Average glucose levels (HbA1c)				
Blood pressure				
Cholesterol level				
Body measurements				
Neck				
Arms				
Chest				
Waist	42 inches	36 inches	-4 inches	2 inches
Hips				
Thighs				
Dress size	16	14	1 size	1 size

Step 3 – Review

Tips:

- Measure yourself in the morning before any food or water. Be consistent with each measurement.
- Be realistic about your goals.

	BEFORE	AFTER	CHANGE	GOAL
Date				
Weight				
Average glucose levels (HbA1c)				
Blood pressure				
Cholesterol level				
Body measurements				
Neck				
Arms				
Chest				
Waist				
Hips				
Thighs				
Dress size				

TRACKING CHARTS

Use the below chart to track your cumulative weight-loss across the weeks. Seeing your progress on the chart shows how far you have come and keeps you motivated.

Use either dates (e.g. January 1st) or days (e.g. day 1, day 2 etc) along the bottom and your own scale along the side (e.g. starting at 180lbs and using 2lb increments). Measure your weight as frequently as you feel comfortable with. Some people like the accountability of measuring every day, while others find it stressful. It is recommended that you measure at least once a week.

The charts can also be used for tracking other metrics. Perhaps track your end of day glucose levels, average GI of the food, calories per day, exercise levels, such as minutes per day walked or your mood – based on a five-point scale. This is all optional but have some fun with it.

Step 3 – Review

WEEKLY PROGRESS

	Week 1	2	3	4	5	6	7	8	9	10	11	12
Weight – Actual	180	175	173	171	170	168	166	166	164	162	160	160
Weight – Change		5	2	2	1	2	2	0	2	2	2	0
Blood Pressure												
Cholesterol Level												
Body Measurements												
Neck												
Arms												
Chest												
Waist	42	40	34.5	34	38.5	38	37.5	37.5	37	36.5	36	36
Hips												
Thighs												

EXAMPLE

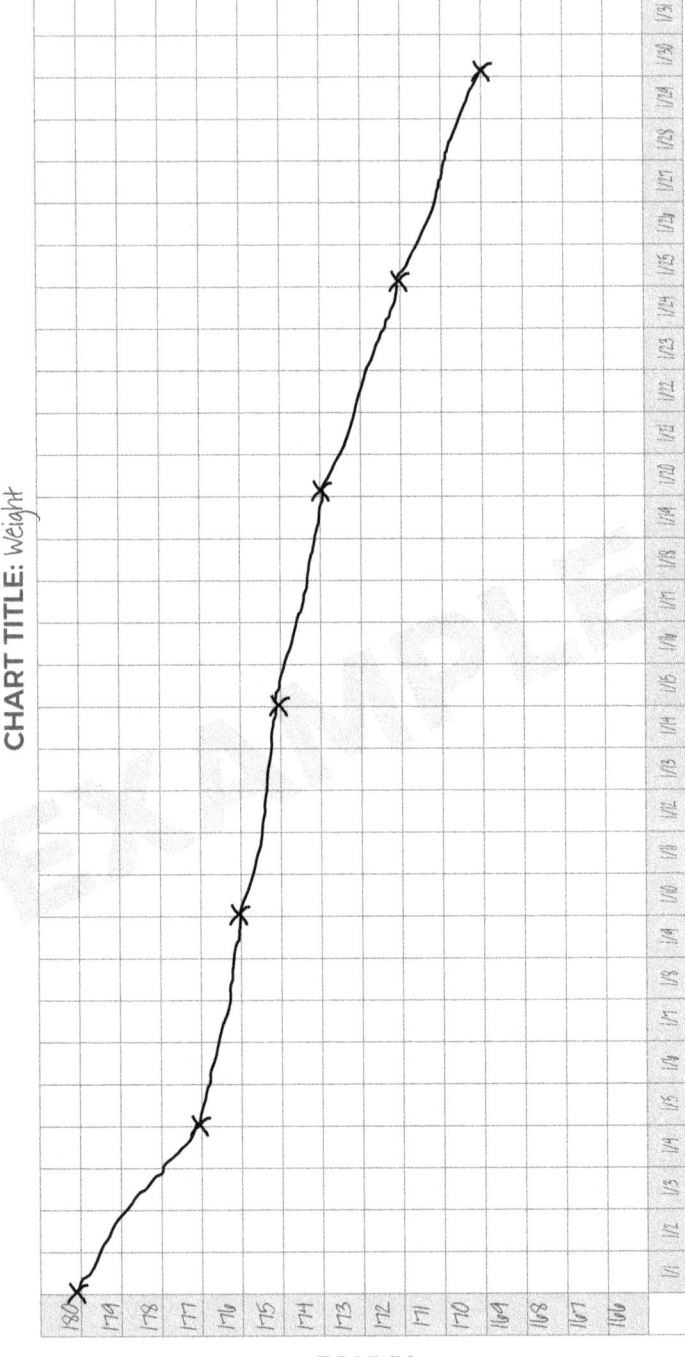

Step 3 – Review

WEEKLY PROGRESS

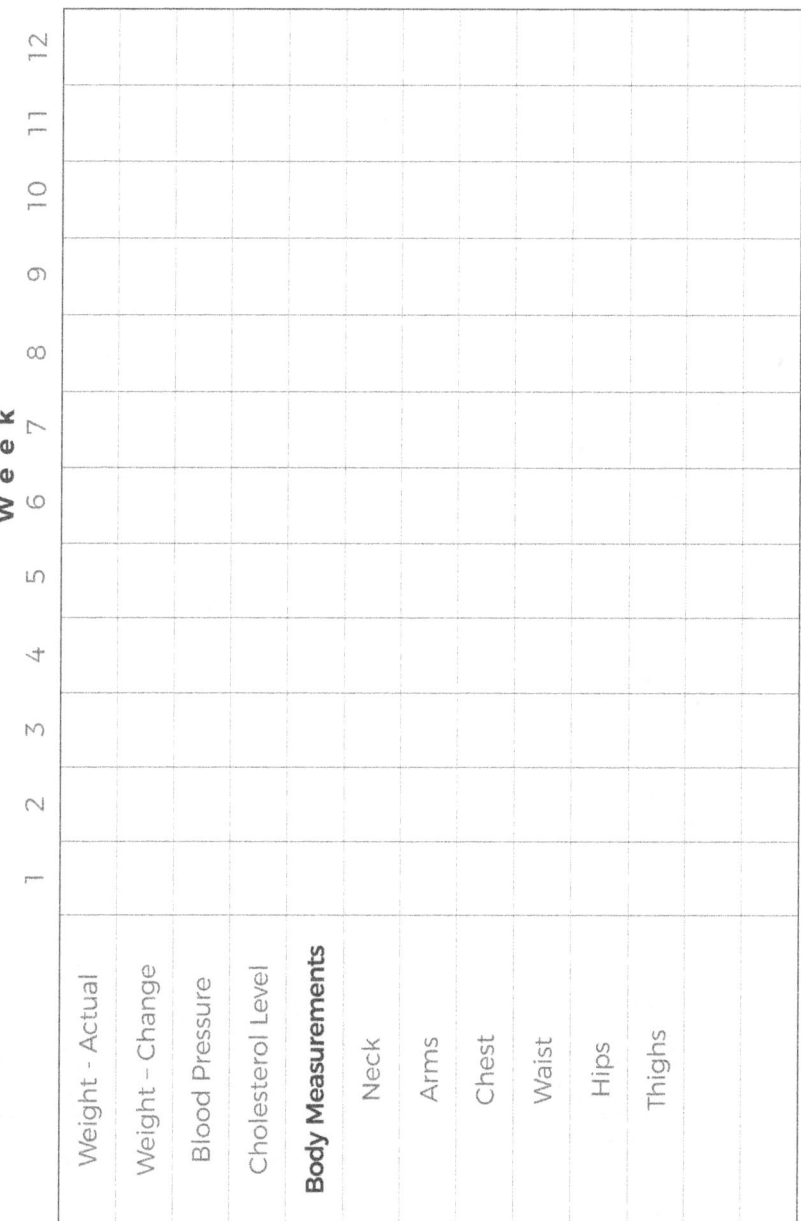

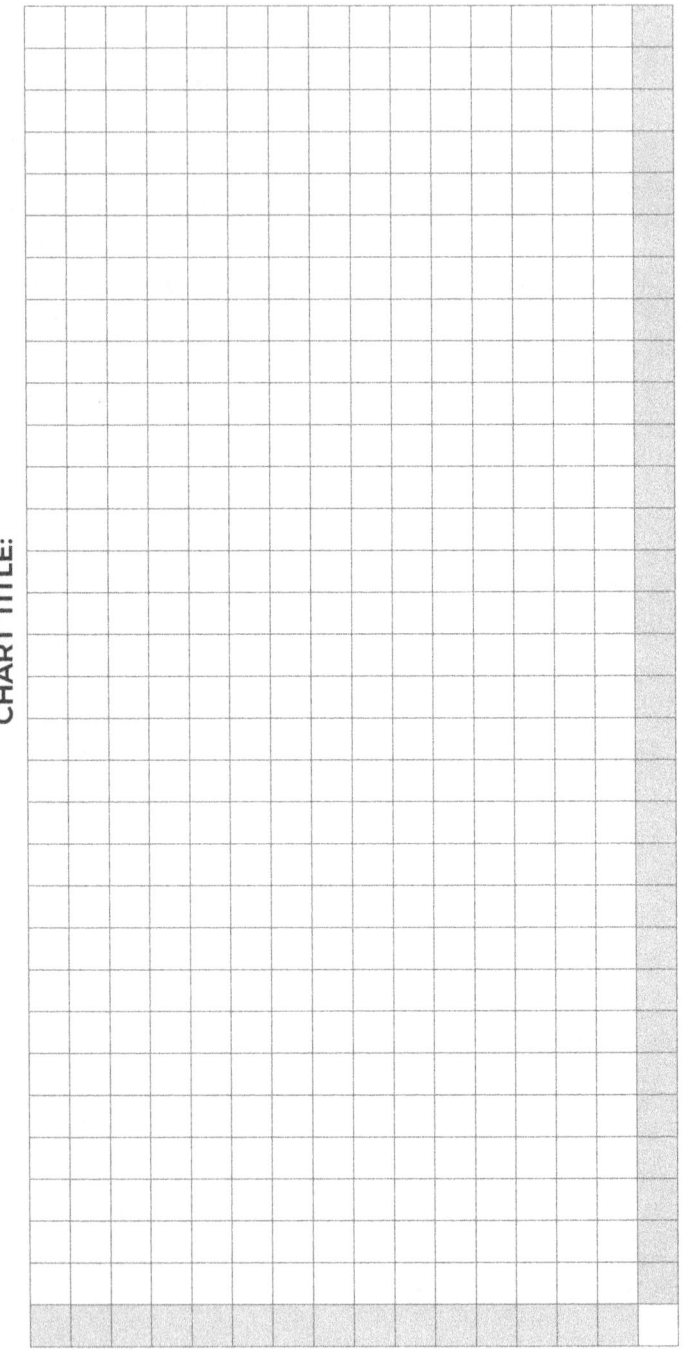

CHART TITLE:

DATE / DAY

RANGE

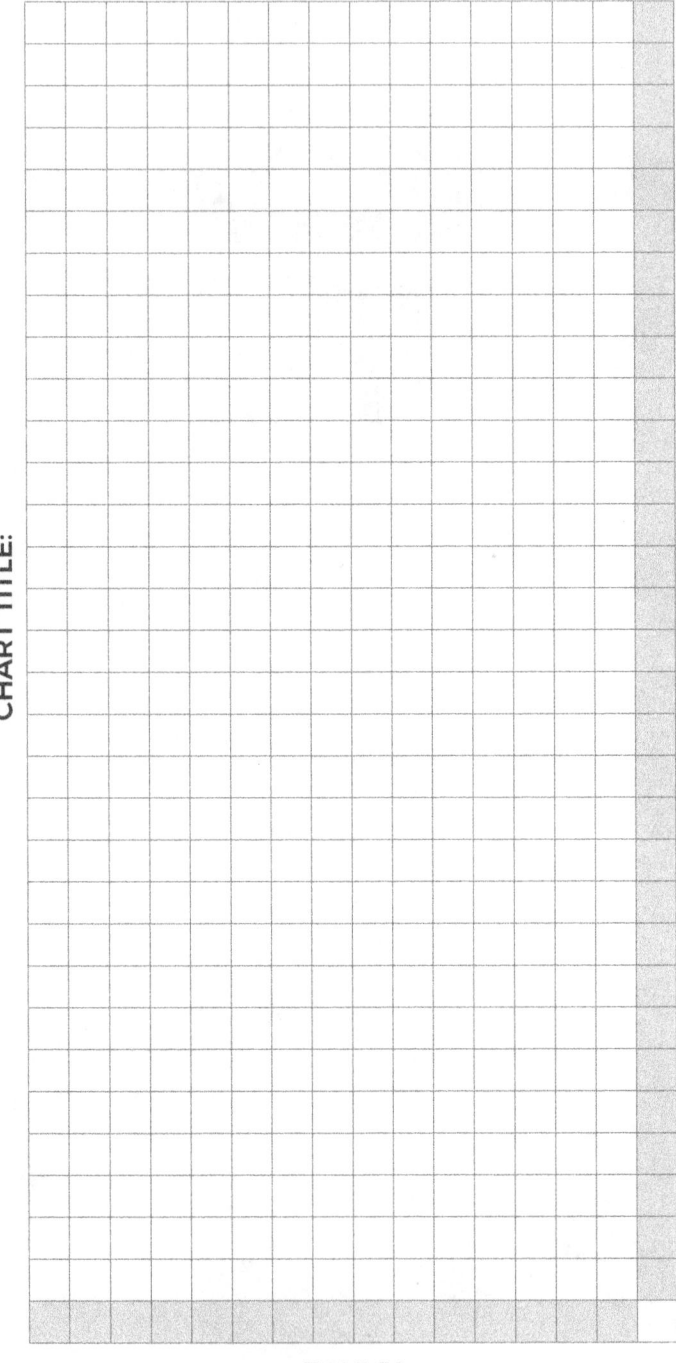

STEP 4
CELEBRATE

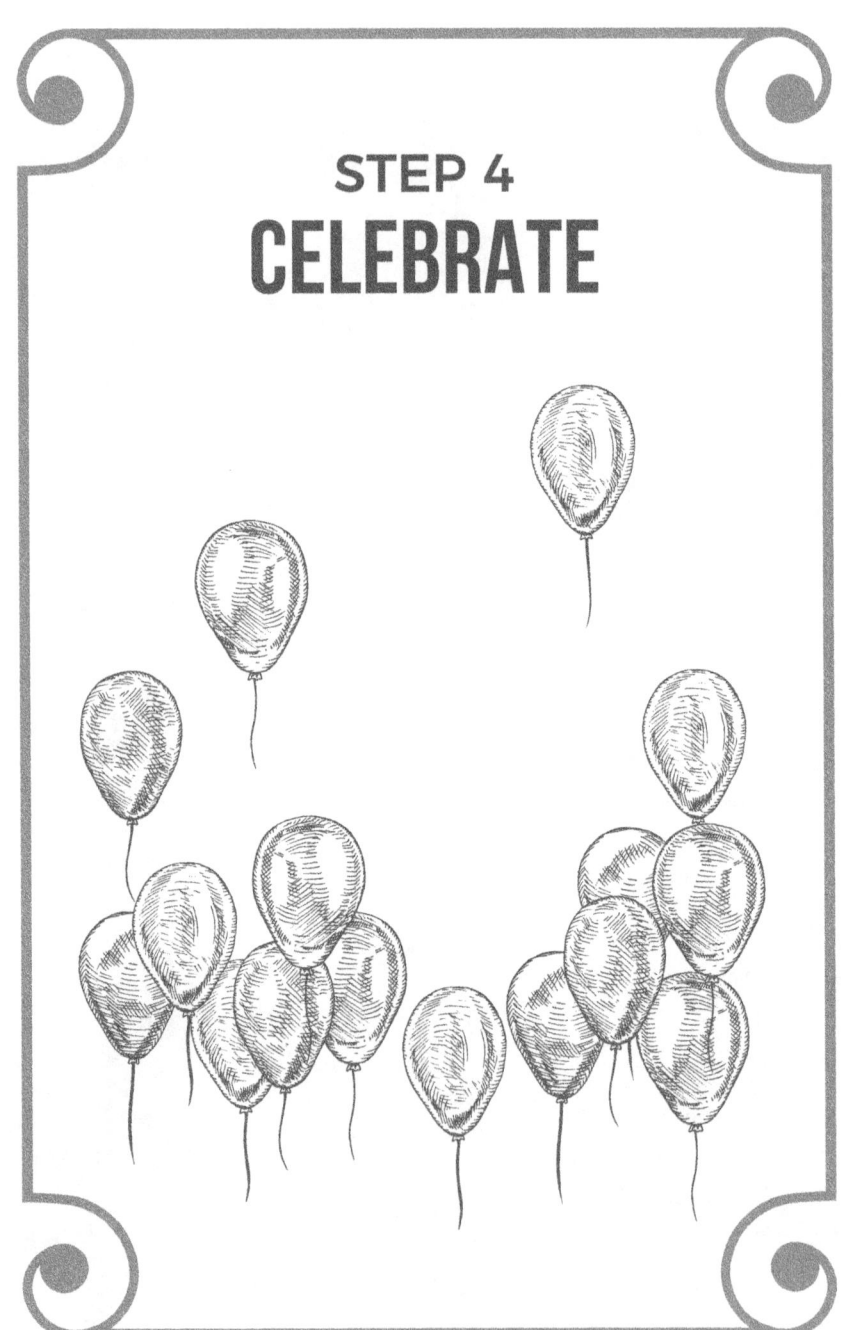

Step 4 – Celebrate

3-MONTH TARGET ACHIEVED

Congratulations – you have achieved three months of tracking your nutrition and working toward your goals. It is definitely time to celebrate.

Whether or not you have achieved your exact goals or have just made progress toward them, I want to sincerely congratulate you and wish you the best for the next steps.

I would invite you to review your journey during the past three months.

- What have you achieved?
- What patterns have emerged?
- What old habits did you have that you can now avoid?
- How can you reinforce your new habits?

I would also love to hear your story and feedback on the process. Please email us at help@habitually-healthy.com and bring a little smile to our faces ☺

Habitually Healthy

> **"IT DOESN'T MATTER HOW FAST OR SLOWLY YOU, SO LONG AS YOU DO NOT STOP"**

APPENDIX

There are several useful reference guides and templates to make the journey easier. Inside you will find:

- Common daily activities and calories burned (some may surprise you).

- A template to record your frequently eaten meals (for easy nutritional reference)

- Recipe notes templates to record your favorite recipes (including ingredients, directions and more)

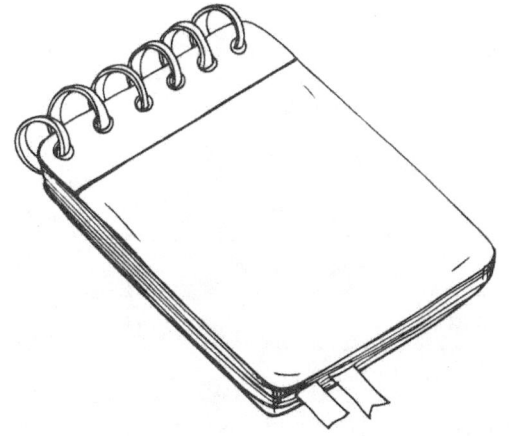

EXERCISE REFERENCE GUIDE

Actual calories burned will vary person to person, dependent on age, gender, metabolism, height, and weight. However, below is a handy list of calories burnt for 30 minutes of activity.

Calories burned in 30-minute activities	
Gym Activities	185-pound person
Aerobics: water	178
Stretching, Hatha yoga	178
Aerobics: low impact	244
Steeper machine: general	266
Aerobics, step: low impact	311
Bicycling, stationary: moderate	311
Rowing, stationary: moderate	311
Training and Sport Activities	
Badminton: general	200
Basketball: general play	355
Bicycling: 12-13.9 mph	355
Dancing: slow, waltz, foxtrot	133
Hiking: cross-country	266
Rope: jumping	444
Running: 5 mph (12 min./mile)	355
Running: 7.5 mph (8 min/mile)	555

Running: 7.5 mph (8 min/mile)	555
Soccer: general	311
Softball: general play	222
Swimming: general	266
Tennis: general	311
Walk/jog: jog <10 min	266
Walking: 4 mph (15 min./mile)	200
Outdoor Activities	
Raking lawn	178
Sacking grass or leaves	178
Gardening: general	200
Dancing: slow, waltz, foxtrot	200
Mowing lawn: push, power	200
Laying sod / crushed rock	222
Mowing lawn: push, hand	244
Home and Daily Life Activities	
Playing with kids: moderate effort	178
Heavy cleaning: wash car, windows	200
Child games: hopscotch, jacks	222
Playing with kids: vigorous effort	222
Moving: household furniture	266
Moving: carrying boxes	311

FREQUENTLY EATEN FOODS

Record your favorite meals for easy reference.

MEALS	Amount	Cal.	Fat gm	Carb. gm	Fiber gm	Sugar gm	Added Sugar gm	Protein gm
Avo' Burger	1 burger	232	20			3		10
Breakfast smoothie	1 glass	178	14			1		12

FREQUENTLY EATEN FOODS

MEALS	Amount	Cal.	Fat gm	Carb. gm	Fiber gm	Sugar gm	Added Sugar gm	Protein gm

RECIPE NOTES

Use this space to record any new favorite recipes you find.

Recipe Name

_____

Ingredients

- _____
- _____
- _____
- _____
- _____
- _____
- _____
- _____
- _____
- _____

Directions

_____
_____
_____
_____
_____
_____
_____
_____
_____
_____
_____
_____

Recommended Occasions

_____
_____

Notes

_____
_____
_____

RECIPE #

Where is the recipe from?
_____

Serves
1   2   3   4   5   6

Prep Time _____:_____
Cook Time _____:_____

Prep Type
_____
_____

Goes Well With
_____
_____

Nutritional Info
Calories _____
Fat _____
Carb _____
Fiber _____
Sugar _____
Added Sugar _____
Protein _____
GI _____

How Tasty?
Difficulty:
1   2   3   4   5
Overall Rating:
😟 😔 😐 🙂 😄

RECIPE NOTES

Use this space to record any new favorite recipes you find.

Recipe Name
_____

Ingredients
- _____
- _____
- _____
- _____
- _____
- _____
- _____
- _____
- _____
- _____

Directions
_____
_____
_____
_____
_____
_____
_____
_____
_____
_____

Recommended Occasions
_____
_____

Notes
_____
_____
_____

RECIPE #

Where is the recipe from?
_____

Serves
1   2   3   4   5   6

Prep Time _____ : _____
Cook Time _____ : _____

Prep Type
_____
_____

Goes Well With
_____
_____

Nutritional Info
Calories _____
Fat _____
Carb _____
Fiber _____
Sugar _____
Added Sugar _____
Protein _____
GI _____

How Tasty?
Difficulty:
1   2   3   4   5
Overall Rating:
😖 😕 😐 🙂 😄

RECIPE NOTES

Use this space to record any new favorite recipes you find.

Recipe Name

Ingredients

-
-
-
-
-
-
-
-
-

Directions

RECIPE #

Where is the recipe from?

Serves
1 2 3 4 5 6

Prep Time _____:_____
Cook Time _____:_____

Prep Type

Goes Well With

Nutritional Info
Calories _____
Fat _____
Carb _____
Fiber _____
Sugar _____
Added Sugar _____
Protein _____
GI _____

Recommended Occasions

Notes

How Tasty?
Difficulty:
1 2 3 4 5
Overall Rating:
😟 😔 😐 🙂 😄

Appendix

RECIPE NOTES

Use this space to record any new favorite recipes you find.

Recipe Name
_____

RECIPE #

Ingredients

- _____   - _____
- _____   - _____
- _____   - _____
- _____   - _____
- _____   - _____
- _____   - _____

Where is the recipe from?
_____

Serves
1   2   3   4   5   6

Prep Time _____ : _____
Cook Time _____ : _____

Prep Type
_____
_____

Directions
_____
_____
_____
_____
_____
_____
_____
_____
_____
_____
_____

Goes Well With
_____
_____

Nutritional Info
Calories _____
Fat   _____
Carb   _____
Fiber   _____
Sugar   _____
Added Sugar _____
Protein   _____
GI _____

Recommended Occasions
_____
_____

Notes
_____
_____
_____

How Tasty?
Difficulty:
1   2   3   4   5
Overall Rating:
😟 😕 😐 🙂 😄

RECIPE NOTES

Use this space to record any new favorite recipes you find.

Recipe Name
_____

Ingredients
- _____ • _____
- _____ • _____
- _____ • _____
- _____ • _____
- _____ • _____

Directions
_____
_____
_____
_____
_____
_____
_____
_____
_____

Recommended Occasions
_____
_____

Notes
_____
_____
_____

RECIPE #

Where is the recipe from?
_____

Serves
1   2   3   4   5   6

Prep Time _____ : _____
Cook Time _____ : _____

Prep Type
_____
_____

Goes Well With
_____
_____

Nutritional Info
Calories _____
Fat _____
Carb _____
Fiber _____
Sugar _____
Added Sugar _____
Protein _____
GI _____

How Tasty?
Difficulty:
1   2   3   4   5
Overall Rating:
😦 😐 🙂 😊 😁

Appendix

RECIPE NOTES

Use this space to record any new favorite recipes you find.

Recipe Name
_____

Ingredients
- _____   - _____
- _____   - _____
- _____   - _____
- _____   - _____
- _____   - _____

Directions
_____
_____
_____
_____
_____
_____
_____
_____
_____

Recommended Occasions
_____
_____

Notes
_____
_____
_____

RECIPE #

Where is the recipe from?
_____

Serves
1 2 3 4 5 6

Prep Time _____
Cook Time _____

Prep Type
_____
_____

Goes Well With
_____
_____

Nutritional Info
Calories _____
Fat _____
Carb _____
Fiber _____
Sugar _____
Added Sugar _____
Protein _____
GI _____

How Tasty?
Difficulty:
1 2 3 4 5
Overall Rating:
☹ 😕 😐 🙂 😄

RECIPE NOTES

Use this space to record any new favorite recipes you find.

Recipe Name
_____

RECIPE #

Ingredients
- _____ - _____
- _____ - _____
- _____ - _____
- _____ - _____
- _____ - _____

Where is the recipe from?
_____

Serves
1   2   3   4   5   6

Prep Time _____ : _____
Cook Time _____ : _____

Prep Type
_____
_____

Directions
_____
_____
_____
_____
_____
_____
_____
_____
_____

Goes Well With
_____
_____

Nutritional Info
Calories _____
Fat _____
Carb _____
Fiber _____
Sugar _____
Added Sugar _____
Protein _____
GI _____

Recommended Occasions
_____
_____

How Tasty?
Difficulty:
1   2   3   4   5

Overall Rating:
😟 😔 😐 🙂 😄

Notes
_____
_____
_____

RECIPE NOTES

Use this space to record any new favorite recipes you find.

Recipe Name
_____

Ingredients
- _____   • _____
- _____   • _____
- _____   • _____
- _____   • _____
- _____   • _____
- _____   • _____

Directions
_____
_____
_____
_____
_____
_____
_____
_____
_____

Recommended Occasions
_____
_____

Notes
_____
_____
_____

RECIPE

Where is the recipe from?
_____

Serves
1   2   3   4   5   6

Prep Time   ____ : ____
Cook Time   ____ : ____

Prep Type
_____
_____

Goes Well With
_____
_____

Nutritional Info
Calories   _____
Fat   _____
Carb   _____
Fiber   _____
Sugar   _____
Added Sugar _____
Protein   _____
GI   _____

How Tasty?
Difficulty:
1   2   3   4   5
Overall Rating:
😖 😕 😐 🙂 😄

RECIPE NOTES

Use this space to record any new favorite recipes you find.

Recipe Name

_____

Ingredients
- _____   • _____
- _____   • _____
- _____   • _____
- _____   • _____
- _____

Directions

_____
_____
_____
_____
_____
_____
_____
_____
_____
_____

Recommended Occasions

_____
_____

Notes

_____
_____
_____

RECIPE #

Where is the recipe from?
_____

Serves
1   2   3   4   5   6

Prep Time _____ : _____
Cook Time _____ : _____

Prep Type
_____
_____

Goes Well With
_____
_____

Nutritional Info
Calories _____
Fat _____
Carb _____
Fiber _____
Sugar _____
Added Sugar _____
Protein _____
GI _____

How Tasty?
Difficulty:
1   2   3   4   5
Overall Rating:
😟 😔 😐 🙂 😄

Appendix

RECIPE NOTES

Use this space to record any new favorite recipes you find.

Recipe Name

_____

Ingredients
- _____   • _____
- _____   • _____
- _____   • _____
- _____   • _____
- _____   • _____
- _____   • _____

Directions

_____
_____
_____
_____
_____
_____
_____
_____

Recommended Occasions

_____
_____

Notes

_____
_____
_____

RECIPE #

Where is the recipe from?
_____

Serves
1   2   3   4   5   6

Prep Time _____ : _____
Cook Time _____ : _____

Prep Type
_____
_____

Goes Well With
_____
_____

Nutritional Info
Calories _____
Fat _____
Carb _____
Fiber _____
Sugar _____
Added Sugar _____
Protein _____
GI _____

How Tasty?
Difficulty:
1   2   3   4   5
Overall Rating:
😟 😕 😐 🙂 😁

Deluxe Diabetes Food & Blood Sugar Journal

RECIPE NOTES

Use this space to record any new favorite recipes you find.

Recipe Name

_____

Ingredients
- _____
- _____
- _____
- _____
- _____
- _____
- _____
- _____
- _____
- _____

Directions

_____
_____
_____
_____
_____
_____
_____
_____

Recommended Occasions

_____
_____

Notes

_____
_____
_____

RECIPE #

Where is the recipe from?
_____

Serves
1   2   3   4   5   6

Prep Time _____ : _____
Cook Time _____ : _____

Prep Type
_____
_____

Goes Well With
_____
_____

Nutritional Info
Calories _____
Fat _____
Carb _____
Fiber _____
Sugar _____
Added Sugar _____
Protein _____
GI _____

How Tasty?
Difficulty:
1   2   3   4   5
Overall Rating:
😖 😕 😐 😊 😁

Appendix

RECIPE NOTES

Use this space to record any new favorite recipes you find.

Recipe Name

_____

Ingredients
- _____
- _____
- _____
- _____
- _____
- _____
- _____
- _____
- _____
- _____

Directions

_____
_____
_____
_____
_____
_____
_____
_____
_____
_____

Recommended Occasions

_____
_____

Notes

_____
_____
_____

RECIPE #

Where is the recipe from?
_____

Serves
1   2   3   4   5   6

Prep Time _____ : _____
Cook Time _____ : _____

Prep Type
_____
_____

Goes Well With
_____
_____

Nutritional Info
Calories _____
Fat   _____
Carb   _____
Fiber   _____
Sugar   _____
Added Sugar _____
Protein   _____
GI   _____

How Tasty?
Difficulty:
1   2   3   4   5
Overall Rating:
☹ 😕 😐 🙂 😄

www.ingramcontent.com/pod-product-compliance
Lightning Source LLC
Chambersburg PA
CBHW031146020426
42333CB00013B/530